◆ FriesenPress

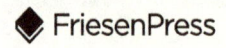

One Printers Way
Altona, MB R0G 0B0
Canada

www.friesenpress.com

Copyright © 2023 by Holly Rae Fehr
First Edition — 2023

Disclaimer: The following information in this book is presented only as a personal opinion and should not in any form replace the medical advice or treatment of a licensed healthcare provider. Always consult a physician for any and all medical advice before attempting any treatments or dietary suggestions mentioned in the book.

All rights reserved.

No part of this publication may be reproduced in any form, or by any means, electronic or mechanical, including photocopying, recording, or any information browsing, storage, or retrieval system, without permission in writing from FriesenPress.

ISBN
978-1-03-917363-7 (Hardcover)
978-1-03-917362-0 (Paperback)
978-1-03-917364-4 (eBook)

1. HEALTH & FITNESS, PREGNANCY & CHILDBIRTH

Distributed to the trade by The Ingram Book Company

Treasured cesarean

The complete, uncensored, healthy mama's guide to accepting, preparing for, and owning your cesarean while healing from the inside out!

Holly Rae Fehr

Illustrated by Abril Dustin

To all of the mamas who are struggling to accept the circumstances of their birth story.

To all of the mamas who have had to find strength that they didn't even know existed.

To all of the mamas who have sat in the closet or on the bathroom floor bawling their eyes out only to open the door up time and time again pretending that everything is okay.

To all of the mamas who keep on showing up day after day for their families, even amongst their own personal struggles and pain that so often goes unnoticed.

You are seen. You are loved and needed more deeply than you know. You are doing the most important work raising your babies. And it is all SO worth it. I promise!

TABLE OF CONTENTS

Chapter 1: Introduction — 3
Who am I? Why did I write this book? And why I think every mom-to-be should prepare for a cesarean even if she is not planning to have one!

Chapter 2: Reasons for a Cesarean Delivery — 9
The more you know, the more you can prepare!

Chapter 3: Owning Your Cesarean — 17
Accepting your birth story and learning to heal from what your expectations were to what your reality has become.

Chapter 4: The Essential Guide to Preparing Your Home for a Cesarean Recovery — 23
What you can do in the days, weeks, and months leading up to your cesarean to make your healing process much easier.

Chapter 5: How to Make the Most of Your Hospital Stay — 41
What to pack in your hospital bags for you, your support partner, and your baby to make the most out of your hospital stay.

Chapter 6: Gentle, Natural, and Family-Centered Birth Plan — 53
Understanding the birthing options that may be available to you even if you are undergoing a cesarean delivery.

Chapter 7: The Day Has Arrived — 61
What to expect the morning of your cesarean and the first few hours after arriving at the hospital.

Chapter 8: It's GO TIME! — 71
What actually happens during surgery and in the recovery room afterwards?

Chapter 9: Timeline for Healing from Your Cesarean — 83
How long until I feel like myself again?

Chapter 10: Breastfeeding — 93
How to overcome the difficulties of breastfeeding while healing from a cesarean.

Chapter 11: NICU Baby — 107
What to expect if your new baby requires time in the NICU after your cesarean

Chapter 12: First Week at Home — 117
Realistic expectations for bringing your baby home during the first week.

Chapter 13: Supplements, Diet, and Exercise for Healing — 127
How to make the most of your pregnancy, cesarean, and postpartum healing through proper nutrition.

Chapter 14: Alternative Therapies for Healing Your Body — 145
What can be done to prevent or heal from long-term complications of a cesarean?

Chapter 15: Role of the Support Partner   **151**
How your support partner can best support you before, during, and after your cesarean.

Chapter 16: Some Final Words   **157**
Encouragement for all cesarean moms

About the Author   **159**

Treasured Cesarean

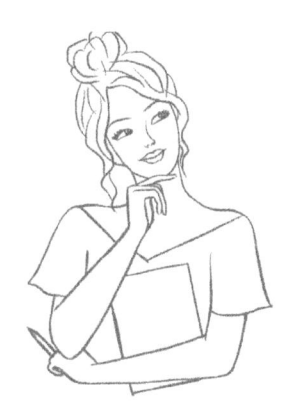

CHAPTER 1
Introduction

Who am I? Why did I write this book? And why I think every mom-to-be should prepare for a cesarean even if she is not planning to have one!

HI! I'M HOLLY RAE. If you currently find yourself reading this book, chances are you might be one of the over 30% of *greatly misrepresented* women who will undergo a cesarean delivery, or maybe you have had one in the past. Maybe you are scared to death because your doctor recently told you a cesarean was the only way to safely deliver your baby, or maybe you have recently had one and are wondering what on earth just happened to your body! You might even be wondering how in your right mind you are going to heal yourself from a major abdominal surgery while caring for your new infant. I get it! That was me over thirteen years and seven cesareans ago.

Like so many newly pregnant mamas, I was completely certain that a cesarean delivery would not be in my cards, not for this mama anyways. After all, I have aways been a natural-minded person and considered myself as someone who was fairly prepared and well informed. If I were completely honest with myself, at the young age of twenty-three, I truly didn't believe C-sections happened to women like me. In fact, I was so certain of this that even while pouring myself into every book and article imaginable about becoming a new mom, I made sure to consistently skip over every single chapter related to cesareans. I was healthy, I was determined, and I was fully prepared for a completely natural delivery… that is, until I wasn't! How naive I was when my water broke only an hour into my official due date—perfectly on time, I thought. Even though I had absolutely no other signs of an impending labor, my bags were packed, I felt amazing, and I was completely excited to meet my new baby boy.

At around 1:00 a.m., while still at home, I cranked up some country music (*no judgement please*) and proceeded to do my makeup and freshen up my hair while my nervous and excited husband started the car and loaded up the bags. It was frigidly cold outside, so we needed to let the vehicle run for a while before we could head out the door. Although I felt a bit anxious, I looked refreshed, felt fantastic, and was completely ready to meet my little baby in the next few hours. Right! (This is the part where it is totally okay to roll your eyes. I honestly had zero clue what was in store for me!) In my innocent, young, and fairly ignorant mind, I had absolutely no idea what the rest of the night and the following day held. We grabbed a coffee on our way in and eagerly headed to the hospital, which was about an hour away from our home.

Once I was admitted, the nurses checked my vitals, monitored my contractions (which were unfortunately pretty much non-existent), and put my husband and me in an observation room. Because we were an hour away from home and the hospital wasn't overly busy that night, we were told we could stay in our room and see how things progressed overnight. Unfortunately, several hours went by and things remained stagnant. It wasn't long before the labor nurse came into the room again and suggested I be induced. Honestly, had I known then what I know now, I would have likely waited much longer before agreeing to an induction. However, my inexperienced self was much more interested in meeting my new baby than waiting for nature to take its course, and I truly believed at the time that since my water had already broken earlier that an induction was the only option.

Although inducing my labor worked wonders to bring on dreadfully strong, painful, and heavy contractions almost immediately, it failed to do anything else. So, there I was, hours and hours into steady and agonizing contractions without any progress at all. Literally nothing. My cervix was refusing to budge! It was *so* deflating and exhausting. I had been in hard labor for over eight hours, and now the day, which had started far before sunrise, was moving into the early evening. As I became increasingly more worn out, the nursing staff brought a monitor into the room to check the baby's vitals again. At that point, I was ready to accept an epidural or pretty much anything else they offered to ease the ongoing contractions that were doing absolutely nothing. As the labor nurse listened to the baby's heartbeat once again, I noticed that her energy was different than before. I saw the look in her countenance become much more worried... *and that was probably the last moment that I can clearly recall in great detail.*

Within moments, the room filled with doctors, nurses, and an anesthesiologist. I remember my husband's eyes looking like a deer caught in the headlights while the hospital staff moved me onto another bed and wheeled me down the hall. They informed me that my little baby's heartbeat was not doing well and that we needed to get the baby out immediately. While on the move, they were giving me all kinds of information and passing me papers to sign even though I was so shaky I could not even clearly see the lines.

Upon entering the operating room, I was hooked up to an IV, given all kinds of information, strapped to a table, and thrown under a blue curtain. The cesarean began before I even had a chance to breathe or contemplate what on earth was going on. I was so scared and emotional, and I truly felt like my baby boy wasn't going to make it out alive. Having had many prior miscarriages, I can remember feeling very alone and hopeless, even though my husband was by my side. I was cold, shaky, and so frightened that I felt like I was going to completely pass out. And then just like that, in what seemed like only a few moments later, my precious baby boy, who almost didn't make it into this world, was placed in my arms. *It was dreadfully perfect.*

Before I get too much further into my story, I want to give you a clear idea of all of the things that I am not. I am not a physician. I am not a naturopathic doctor. I am not a nurse. I am also not living in your specific shoes, and therefore, I am unable to tell you exactly what you should do and what choices will be the best for you and your family. Those are very personal decisions that will take much reflection and discussion with your partner and your medical team. I am, however, the mother of seven beautiful children on Earth and ten angel babies in Heaven. All of my Earthly babies were beautifully introduced to this world through cesarean delivery rather than vaginally. That's right! I have had seven cesareans, each one wildly unique and personal in its own way. Although my first cesarean definitely caught me fiercely by surprise (and as mentioned above, I was not the least bit prepared), the following six births were all planned, repeat cesareans... *and I loved every one of them!*

A question I am often asked is, "Do you regret having chosen a repeat cesarean now that you have had seven babies?" Here is my most common response:

Knowing now what I did not know many years ago, I do think I would have likely chosen to attempt a VBAC (vaginal birth after cesarean), and I do wish I had researched labor and delivery—including cesareans—prior to giving birth for the first time. I do believe that a natural vaginal birth is always the healthiest option both for mom and baby, and I will always wonder what things would have been different if I had tried harder for a vaginal delivery. However, not for one single moment have I ever regretted the way my babies were brought into this world! Each one arrived in their own unique way and has their own special story to accompany their births. Each precious baby was placed into my arms and immediately filled me with an overwhelming love that instantly permeated the moment with awe-struck feelings of joy. I don't feel for one small moment less of a mother or a woman because of the way my babies arrived. I am thankful for each and every birth story and have chosen to be joyous and content regardless of their type of delivery!

I also want to be very clear about what you can and cannot expect from reading this book. If you are looking for a basic, long, drawn-out version of the hospital pamphlets they send you home with after your surgery, you will not find that here. If you want to find out all of the statistics or scare tactics your friends have probably already informed you of regarding the benefits of vaginal delivery versus cesarean delivery, you will definitely not find that in this book either. If you are looking for advice as to whether or not you should have a repeat cesarean or attempt a VBAC, you will again not find that information anywhere in this book. That is a decision that should not be taken lightly and should be discussed with your doctors while also taking time to reflect on what is best for you. (Many amazing books have already been written that will give you insight into natural birth options, ways to improve your chances of having a VBAC, and many other topics. I highly recommend you dig into them before you make any major decisions.) In fact, if you get even a tiny bit of any of the ideas listed above after reading this book, then I have definitely failed to convey my heart to you.

You see, my goal is not to shame or frighten you, but rather to encourage you, strengthen you, and prepare you for whatever situation you find yourself in. It is none of my business, nor anyone else's for that matter, why you might undergo a cesarean (whether it's your first time or perhaps a repeat), or even if you are healing from an emergency C-section. I am not here to play the guilt game that is so popular among so many mothers and well-meaning friends (and unfortunately, even complete strangers) with you. I want to familiarize you with what the process is truly like, from one mom to another. I want to share with you all of the unique strategies I have learned over time in hopes that you can use them to better prepare for your cesarean and truly heal from the inside out. And I desperately want you to not only accept your cesarean delivery, but fully cherish your beautiful birth story—every last detail of it.

It is also my hope that this book will change the perspective of women everywhere who find themselves undergoing a cesarean delivery. You have every bit as much of a reason to feel valued with your birth story, even when you are sitting with the circle of mamas at the coffee shop making small talk about your babies. Just because your birth did not end up as you were hoping does not make you a failure or any less worthy. In fact you are strong, capable, and every bit qualified as a mom, regardless of how your baby was or will be delivered. You did nothing wrong. Rather, you did what was needed to be done or will do what is necessary to bring your child into this world. You've got this, Mama!

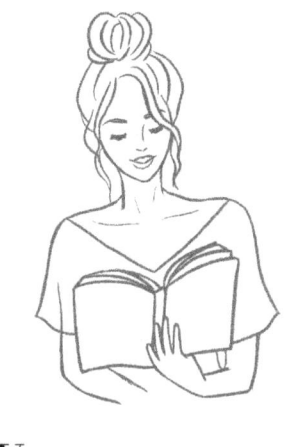

CHAPTER 2
Reasons for a Cesarean Delivery

The more you know, the more you can prepare!

BEFORE I GET to the exciting part of the book, I want to quickly cover some of the basic reasons why a mom-to-be may end up requiring a cesarean, even if it is completely not part of her game plan. Even if you fully believe you will have a vaginal delivery—like I did—it is a good idea to familiarize yourself with these various scenarios to make things less of a surprise should you find yourself in any of the situations described. This chapter is not meant to scare you at all, but rather to inform you. Childbirth is a major event, and the more you know in advance, the better suited you can be to prevent, or at least prepare for, anything that should come your way.

"While failing to prepare, you are preparing to fail."
—Benjamin Franklin

According to americanpregnancy.org,[1] there are several reasons why a woman may end up having a cesarean. Although some women choose an elective cesarean without having any medical reason for it, most cesareans either occur in critical situations or to prevent a critical situation. In 2020, the CDC stated that 31.8% of all deliveries in the US were cesarean, while Canada followed closely behind at 29.1%.[2] *That is almost one third of all births*—another reason why it is so good to be well researched and prepared.

Reason #1
Failure to Progress

Many things can cause labor to slow down or stop altogether, such as the size of the baby's head, the position of the baby, inefficient contractions, or having a cervix that is not dilating fast enough. More often than not, "failure to progress" is diagnosed during the second part of labor since the first part of labor typically progresses at a much slower rate. All too commonly, healthcare professionals choose a cesarean as a first resort, and if you are not well prepared, you may be eager to give in to their recommendations much too early in the birthing progress. If there is one area that I wish I had been more knowledgeable in with my first child, it would have been this: knowing that labor and delivery is not a sprint; it's a marathon. However, if your body is saying that enough is enough, or your medical team is insistent that the safest route for mom and baby is to move towards a cesarean, then by all means go with it. Feel free to grieve at that moment. In fact, it is completely normal and part of the healing process

---

[1] https://americanpregnancy.org/healthy-pregnancy/labor-and-birth/reasons-for-a-cesarean/
[2] https://pubmed.ncbi.nlm.nih.gov/31883751/

to undo your expectations in exchange for something you were not hoping for. Just be sure to also be present and excited for the fast-approaching arrival of your treasured little bundle. Soon you will be holding your little baby in your arms and everything else beforehand will seem like a blur.

Reason #2
Carrying Multiple Babies

If you are one of those mamas who are carrying multiples and your babies are not positioned properly, you may be more likely to have a cesarean. Whether it is an emergency or planned, you may find yourself quickly preparing for your C-section. On the contrary, I also know of many moms who had both of their twin babies vaginally. This is another scenario where careful planning, preparation, and discussions with your medical team are of most importance.

There are definitely things you can do to increase the chances of a vaginal delivery if you are carrying multiple babies, and by all means take the time to research all of the options available to you. If you are carrying triplets or more, it is much more likely that you will be preparing for a cesarean. Sometimes, there will also be the scenario where one of the babies is delivered vaginally only to have their twin delivered by cesarean. *God bless those mamas' hearts!* That is an entirely new level of healing. Regardless of where you specifically find yourself within the options listed above, being prepared for a cesarean delivery when carrying multiples is always a good idea.

Reason #3
Previous Cesarean

It is completely possible to have a vaginal birth after a cesarean, and it's even possible to attempt a vaginal birth after two cesareans (although you might have trouble finding a practitioner who is willing to take that on). If you are willing to try that, I would definitely take the time to research OB/GYNs in your area and even be willing to drive a little if you want to find one who is encouraging and comfortable to work with. However, many women either choose to avoid a repeat emergency cesarean as needed with a previous baby, or they find themselves going for a repeat after hours of an attempted second vaginal delivery. If this is you, regardless of how you came to this situation, it is totally OKAY! Both you and your baby are going to be okay, and there are SO many things you can do to help yourself heal, both emotionally and physically.

Reason #4
Cord Prolapse

Although rare, a cord prolapse is when the baby's umbilical cord slips into the vagina where there is a likely chance that it will be flattened or squeezed during a vaginal birth. This actually happened to my sister, and she was only seconds away from requiring a very scary, emergency cesarean if not for her amazing doctor doing some pretty quick thinking to get the baby out! Because the umbilical cord is responsible for carrying food and oxygen from the placenta to the baby, this can very quickly escalate into an intense moment for both mom and baby. Although not all cord prolapses will end up in an emergency cesarean, most will. If you find yourself in this situation, stay calm knowing that your medical team is prepared for these scenarios, and they are definitely experienced in providing you with the safest outcome.

Reason # 5
Abnormal Position of the Baby

The ideal birth position of a baby is head down, also known as cephalic presentation. Sometimes, babies will have their own ideas as to how they want to spend their time in-utero. They may be lying in a breech position where his or her bottom or feet are facing down, or in a transverse position where a shoulder is facing down. Often babies will turn around as they approach their due date. However, if your little baby insists on remaining in one of those positions, a cesarean delivery may be in everyone's best interest.

Reason # 6
Placenta Previa

About one in every two hundred pregnant women will experience placenta previa during the third trimester. This is a condition where the placenta lies low in the uterus and partially or fully covers the cervix. Depending on the degree of severity, the doctor may advise bed rest and frequent monitoring if this condition is detected. Placenta previa can be complete, partial, or marginal. If a marginal placenta previa has been diagnosed, a vaginal delivery may still be an option for you and your baby. This is because as the uterus grows and stretches over time, it will likely create more distance between the placenta and the cervix. However, if a complete or partial placenta previa has been diagnosed, a cesarean will likely be recommended.

Reason # 7
Fetal Distress

Although fairly rare, fetal distress is another complication of labor. If the baby does not get enough oxygen during delivery, it experiences distress requiring an emergency C-section to deliver the baby safely. Causes for this could be due to a very difficult labor or if the pregnancy extends itself past forty-two weeks and the baby shows signs of distress. Please note that many babies are perfectly fine to wait slightly past forty-two weeks. Unfortunately, some OB/GYNs do not want to have a woman continue their pregnancy past forty-two weeks and will automatically recommend either inducing you or a cesarean. Make sure that you discuss your options and your desires with your medical team well in advance. As long as the baby is continuing to do well, you may be a great candidate to wait just a while longer for labor to begin on its own!

Reason # 8
Uterine Rupture

One in approximately 1,500 women experience a condition called uterine rupture, and this will require an emergency cesarean. Uterine rupture occurs when the uterus tears during pregnancy or labor and causes hemorrhaging, which then interferes with the baby's supply of oxygen. In these situations, an emergency cesarean is the only possible option for delivery.

Reason # 9
Chronic Health Conditions

Women who suffer from chronic health conditions may be advised to have their baby delivered by cesarean. These chronic conditions could range from gestational diabetes to heart disease to high blood pressure, or something in between. Vaginal delivery with one of these conditions may be dangerous for the mother-to-be depending on the severity of the particular situation. If the mama-to-be has any infections such as genital herpes or HIV that could be transferred to the baby through vaginal delivery, cesarean section is also generally performed.

Reason # 10
Cephalopelvic Disproportion (also known as CPD)

This is a condition where the baby's head is too large to pass through the birth canal, or the mother's cervix is too small for the baby to pass through. This scenario will often lead to a cesarean delivery.

Delivering a baby is no walk in the park, and labor and delivery can be completely unpredictable, no matter how prepared you are in advance. It is absolutely best to prepare yourself for any possible situation so that you can feel empowered once your baby is ready to make his or her grand appearance into this world. I guarantee there are many new moms who found themselves suddenly having a C-section without ever thinking that this would happen to them. Knowing in advance that these things do happen to women of all ages and from all walks of life will help you to accept your circumstances and thrive with your birth story, regardless of the outcome.

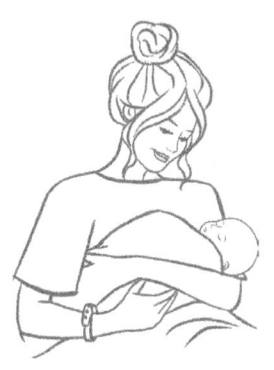

CHAPTER 3
Owning Your Cesarean

Accepting your birth story and learning
to heal from what your expectations were
to what your reality has become.

OKAY! Now that we have covered all of our bases as to why you are preparing for or healing from a cesarean, we can move on to accepting your birth story and choosing to *own* your particular circumstances and flourish. In order to flourish with the birth of your child, you may need to deal with the guilt and disappointment that sometimes accompanies the loss of the opportunity to have a vaginal delivery. *I know I did.* If you do not have guilt or disappointment, that is totally okay, too! Feel free to skip through this section. However, even if you are not having these feelings, I encourage you to read through this chapter with an open mind. You never know when you may be able to lift up another mom who might be struggling simply by sharing your experiences with her.

First off, let's get to a place of understanding that having a cesarean is still giving birth! Birth is birth regardless of how your baby enters this world. I think part of the disappointment with delivering a baby through cesarean is simply the way we as a society have defined this type of delivery. Let's take a look at the following two definitions:

Cesarean delivery: *Also called Cesarean section. Informal: C-section. An operation by which a fetus is taken from the uterus by cutting through the walls of the abdomen and uterus.* Yikes! That doesn't sound all that beautiful or encouraging, does it?

Birth: *an act or instance of bringing forth a child.*

Much better! That is the way we are supposed to view bringing a baby into this world. But so often we automatically assume that *birth* only refers to a vaginal delivery, while a cesarean is simply a cold, mechanical procedure for getting a baby out.

To be honest, I was completely flabbergasted when I read these definitions side by side. When we as a society separate the term *birth* from *cesarean* or *C-section*, we are instantly labelling one scenario as *bringing forth a child* and the other as *cutting out a fetus*! Wow! How unfair is that? We undermine the fact that how a baby enters this world (through our vaginas or through our bellies) makes absolutely no difference as to how they were *birthed*. We need to make sure we are not mislabeling a mother simply by matter of circumstance. No wonder we feel deflated when we have to tell friends and family that our entire pregnancy ended up as a *cesarean* rather than the vaginal birth we were secretly hoping and praying for.

If we continue to view *cesarean* as a stone-cold procedure for delivering a baby, we will never reach the point of understanding cesarean deliveries in the right light. You are simply not *less worthy* than any other mamas who have given birth to a baby vaginally. For the last nine months, you carried your baby and dreamt about your baby just like that other mom. And just like any other mom, you will get to hold and bond with your precious baby as soon as they place him or her into your arms. When your baby first looks into your eyes, he will instantly know the depth of love that you have for him regardless of how he made his grand appearance. And when your baby grows up, you can share with him how you were filled with joy the minute you held him in your arms and how you found the strength within yourself to take care of his needs, even amongst all the challenges that came with healing from a surgery! This is definitely something to be extremely proud of!

After my first son was born by emergency cesarean, I could not believe the number of friends and family who would say things like, "I'm sorry it ended up in a cesarean!" or "Hopefully next time things will work out better!" I even had one acquaintance suggest that *had I avoided being induced, I would have likely had the vaginal delivery I was so highly anticipating!* Whether this was true or not was completely irrelevant. There are things that should *never*, *EVER* be said when a mom has just given birth. (Please, for the sake of new moms everywhere, remember this when friends or family have babies, too!)

I can remember being so disappointed, tired, emotionally drained, and completely inexperienced as to how to heal from my surgery while being solely responsible for taking care of this new little infant in my arms. All I wanted and needed was encouragement and excitement from others for my new arrival. Unfortunately, that's not always the case. Although you cannot avoid all of the negativity or interesting things people will say, you can choose to ignore those comments, shake the dust off your feet, and move forward. Only you know the emotional rollercoaster you and your baby have just been through, and regardless of how you got there, you are probably holding your amazingly perfect little baby in your arms, doting over their every movement. Don't let anyone take those precious first moments from you. You absolutely do not need to accept that negativity as part of your story. Decide ahead of time that regardless of how your baby is born, you will choose to be a positive light for you and your baby.

We need to get past the belief that a cesarean is a second-rate birth option because, more often than not, the women put in this position didn't have a choice in the outcome. I find we as a society tend to view giving birth like the 100-metre dash we all had to run in elementary school:

- All-natural home birth—1st place red ribbon
  - All-natural hospital birth—2nd place blue ribbon
    - Vaginal delivery at the hospital—3rd place green ribbon
      - Cesarean delivery—purple participation ribbon. Thanks for trying!

You see, labor and delivery are just so much more than a series of events. They're about you, the mother, bringing a new life into the world that you have just spent the last nine months caring for. It's about the strength you have within yourself to bring a new little soul into fruition, a tiny baby who, regardless of the birthing outcomes, relies solely on you—his or her mother—to sustain their life. If we continue to devalue cesarean births as a second-rate birth option, we are only doing ourselves a disfavor by not valuing our experiences for what they really are: the ability to become a mom!

Luckily, alongside some quirky and, frankly, quite rude comments, I was also surrounded by many family members and close friends who were beyond amazing—and you will likely be too. These are your people! These are the people you need to surround yourself with as a new mother. These are the people who will walk with you through the healing process. These are the people you should not hesitate to ask for help or simply talk to about your experiences, needs, and emotions.

You are a warrior, Mama! Don't let anyone or any predisposed way of thinking steal that from you. Enjoy this time getting to know your new baby, and don't worry about what others may think or say.

CHAPTER 4
The Essential Guide to Preparing Your Home for a Cesarean Recovery

What you can do in the days, weeks, and months leading up to your cesarean to make your healing process much easier.

REGARDLESS OF whether or not you end up having a vaginal or cesarean delivery, you will definitely want to start preparing your home in advance. Luckily, most pregnancies naturally come with a "nesting period," which is simply the time when a mom-to-be gets the urge to clean, organize, prepare food, and get all things in order before the arrival of the baby. If this is not your first baby, you will likely have experienced this before. If you are planning for a cesarean delivery, there are even more things you can do in and around your home to make it a much more pleasant experience when you bring your baby home. Even if, like me, you are *assuming* you will have an uneventful, natural delivery, it doesn't hurt to do a few little extras just in case.

If your cesarean is planned in advance, you will likely get a date for your surgery sometime during the last trimester. Sometimes, your doctor will choose to wait until closer to your due date to schedule your surgery, while other times they will book it much further in advance. I have experienced both of these scenarios. It really just depends on your body, your baby, and the specifics of your pregnancy. If you are planning for a vaginal delivery, but you're still reading this book, it is safe to assume that you are simply taking extra precautions so you are ready to take on anything that comes your way. In that case, you likely do not know the exact date your baby will arrive. If you do end up with a cesarean, it will most likely be an emergency, at which point it is even more important to be extra prepared when it comes to having a baby!

Because I was so caught off guard with my first cesarean, I did not have anything in place at home to make the situation easier when I was discharged from the hospital. Unfortunately for me, this meant that only ten days after bringing my baby home, I ended up returning to the hospital with a leaking incision, intense abdominal pain, a high fever, and then needing to have an intravenous placed in my arm to administer antibiotics for a severe infection. Because I did not have a clue how to properly heal my body, my incision had opened up after I attempted to do way too many things while caring for my new baby, including saving my brother-in-law from a charging bull. (More on that later!)

Sure, they send you home with a few pamphlets and a quick rundown of what to expect, but I did not find this at all sufficient for the realities of what it was really like to heal, such as: *When will I stop bleeding from my vagina? How much, if at all, should my incision leak? How do I know if I am doing too much?*

Mixed in with the anxiety about my body healing correctly were other concerns that filled my mind: *What if my baby is up night after night, and it's more than I am capable of? What about my bowel movements? I am getting so bloated and still do not feel like I can use the bathroom properly! I have an appointment and my husband has to go back to work soon, is it okay to drive just this one time? I have absolutely no time for myself! How can I feed my baby if I can't even take care of myself?*

I was definitely not planning to leave the hospital in this much pain and was completely confused and overwhelmed with what the next few days, weeks, and even months would hold. What was this really going to be like?

Even though healing officially starts from the moment your baby is born, there are so many extra steps you can do in advance to allow yourself the best possible outcome for bringing your baby home. From organizing your home, packing your bags with cesarean essentials, and choosing to eat a nutritious diet that encourages healing, using the last trimester to set yourself up for success is well worth the effort; take my word for it! It goes without being said that in all of my future pregnancies, I made sure I was much more prepared!

Getting ready for the arrival of a new baby requires a lot of preparation and organization, no matter which way your baby arrives. However, with a cesarean, there are many additional things you can do in advance to make it much easier on you and your family while you heal from your surgery. Below I have shared my "go-to" checklists that I absolutely cannot live without when preparing for a new baby. Although you will see many similarities to preparing for a vaginal delivery, each list contains tips and ideas specifically created for your cesarean. Enjoy!

At-Home Breastfeeding, Pumping, and Changing Essentials

The number-one area where you will want to be extremely organized when bringing a baby home after a cesarean is your feeding and changing stations. You should have *two* carefully laid-out feeding and changing stations for you and your baby: one in the bedroom where your baby will sleep and the other in the main area of the home. This is separate from the nursery you likely have so perfectly arranged. You'll be able to transition into the nursery room soon enough, but during the few days or even weeks immediately following your surgery, you will want these spaces closer to where you'll spend the most of your time.

Let's start with the bedroom feeding and changing station. If at all possible, I highly recommend having the baby sleep in your bedroom—in a separate bassinet, playpen, or crib—for at least the first several weeks until your body has started to recover well. All of my babies remained in my room for their first four to six months; however, this is a timeframe that is completely up to you. I usually moved them into their own rooms once I noticed them becoming more aware of our movements and more likely to wake up when my husband or I entered the room. Having them in a bed close to you is *so* important while you are healing from your cesarean because it allows you to feed and care for them throughout the night without having to move from one room to another.

Walking around with an incision while you are tired and caring for an infant can be physically draining at times. The more streamlined all of your supplies are and the closer you are to your baby, the easier it will be to stay rested while you are doing their night feedings. Ideally, if you can have your baby situated at a similar height as your bed, it will be easier for you to reach over and pick them up for feeding them and changing their diapers as needed (especially in the middle of the night). If you are using a playpen, most of them will come with a bassinet insert that you can use to prevent yourself from having to bend down low to pick up the baby, especially during the first week or two.

If your bed is higher up and your baby is not directly beside you, you may also find it useful to have a small step stool to help you climb on and off the bed for the first few days you are home. Even movements like moving in and out of bed or having to reach too far can be tricky in the early days. After the birth of my fifth baby, it felt as though one of my nerves was pinched in my abdomen, likely from one of my internal stitches. It was an excruciating pain that I had not ever experienced before. There was one particular motion with my left leg that I could not make without feeling a searing pain jolt down my entire body. Although the pain only lasted for a few days, having a stool beside my bed made all of the difference at the time. It never hurts to be extra prepared.

Feeding and Changing Station Checklist

You should have the following supplies easily accessible within reaching limits of your bed:

- ☐ Nursing pads
- ☐ A spare nursing bra and shirt should you leak through in the night
- ☐ All of your pumping supplies if you are planning to pump at all
- ☐ Oversized water bottle (you will likely be very, very thirsty)
- ☐ Simple snacks so that you can take your medication with something in your stomach
- ☐ Lip gloss
- ☐ Burp cloths
- ☐ Diapers and wipes
- ☐ Natural diaper cream
- ☐ Several changes of sleepers for your baby
- ☐ Receiving blankets
- ☐ Phone charger
- ☐ Your phone
- ☐ A safe place to store your vitamins and pain medication
- ☐ A pen and paper or phone app to track what time you took your medication
- ☐ A soother if you are planning to use one with your baby

Now that you have your bedroom ready to go, you should create a similar setup in the main area of your home. Fitting all your supplies in an easy-to-move basket (no more than two) is even more ideal. This way, your support partner or other friends and family can easily move your supplies for you when you transition to different areas of the house. (Remember to keep your medication up high or in a safe place if you have little people running around!) You also want to be sure you are set up close to a comfortable chair—optimally one that reclines or has extra cushions for resting.

When it comes to the baby sleeping during the day, I always kept a small bassinet in the kitchen for my baby to sleep in. This allowed me to not have to move all over the house when they woke throughout the day. When your baby is so young, you really don't need to worry about throwing them out of routine by having them sleep in a different bed during the day than at night. To be honest, I actually found that having them sleep in the main living area during the day and the bedroom at night helped them sort out any day/night confusion very quickly. As soon as you're healed up, you can focus on transitioning all of their sleeps into the same place, but for now, you want to ensure that your healing comes first. It doesn't matter if you use a playpen or a bassinet as their day bed. What matters now is that your baby has a cozy place to lay their head during the day that is in close proximity to you. You won't want to wander long distances to take care of their needs.

> **Quick Tip:** If you do have steps that you have to go up and down often, walk backwards up them! I know it sounds crazy, but it actually allows you to use your back and leg muscles more than your front stomach muscles while they are healing and tender, and it can prevent a lot of pain. Even if you only do this for the first few days, it will make a huge difference long term!

Bathroom Essentials

You'll also want a few specific items in all of the bathrooms you plan on using during your recovery. Depending on the layout of your house, this may mean that you only need to properly stock one bathroom, but perhaps in your situation you may have two or more that you'll want to stock. Whichever bathrooms you believe will be most commonly used during healing should be the ones you focus on.

Because postpartum bleeding after a cesarean can continue up to six weeks or more after delivery (yes, you still bleed after cesarean delivery), you'll want to be stocked up on pads—and not just one size! I highly recommend purchasing some of the biggest ones you can find as well as several other sizes you can easily adjust depending on your flow. Because your uterus contracts and shrinks every time you breastfeed, you should be prepared for larger gushes of blood after each feeding. This is completely normal, but it can come as an uncomfortable surprise if you are not prepared. Also, if you have been sitting or lying down for longer periods of time, your flow can change rapidly again. It's important to have pads and extra panties available in case you need a quick change.

Another important item to have is a natural nipple cream. If you have it in the bathroom, you can easily apply it after your showers or as needed to prevent cracked nipples. Be mindful of the ones you can purchase at the drugstore; although they might say they are safe for baby, some still contain chemicals that I am not overly comfortable having my baby digest. If you only purchase one bottle of nipple cream, you'll probably want to first store it in your hospital bag, and then relocate it to your bathroom after you arrive home. Another great option is to use colloidal silver gel, which also acts as a natural antibiotic. This actually saved me during all of my future cesareans, and you will hear me rave more about it later!

Even though you probably have a good supply of nursing pads in your bedroom and/or main area of the house, having a few extra in the bathroom is not a bad idea either. This way you can easily insert them immediately after your shower. Once your milk comes in, you never know when you will have surprises or leaky breasts. It is always good to have an extra layer of protection.

You should also make sure you have a stack of separate towelettes that you can use to pat the area around your incision dry, especially after you have a shower. This will go a long way in keeping your incision site clean and preventing an infection.

Have some soft bath towels clean and ready to go in the bathroom where you'll shower. Trust me, the extra effort it takes to walk to the laundry room or to the linen closet after all of the effort you have already put into showering your body is exhausting and can totally be avoided. Keep an extra set of laundry fresh and ready to go just in case you end up going into the hospital earlier than expected.

As I've already mentioned, you definitely want to have colloidal silver gel stocked in your bathroom. It makes an amazing antibacterial nipple cream, and it also does wonders when applied directly over your incision. Because cesarean moms are much more prone to infection, this can go a long way in protecting you and your incision. Not only can it help to prevent bacteria from entering your incision area, but it can also assist with healing your incision at a much faster rate and feels wonderful when applied. I always started applying this from the first few days after I had my surgery and continued to do so until I felt as though the cesarean was closed up well and healed thoroughly.

Of course, having some new, basic makeup essentials on hand as well as some hair ties can help you feel fresh and can brighten you up. Even if you are not expecting a lot of company, it might feel nice to have a new mascara, lip gloss, and cheek color just to perk yourself up a little! And if adding makeup is the last thing on your mind or is something that is entirely not important to you, that is obviously okay too!

It is also SO important to have a glass of water or a full water bottle nearby at all times. Even the strenuous motion of showering can easily make you feel dehydrated. It is always good to keep easy access to water all over the house.

Bathroom Checklist

- ☐ Pads of various sizes
- ☐ Extra underwear
- ☐ Natural nipple cream
- ☐ Nursing pads
- ☐ Separate towelettes
- ☐ Fresh towels
- ☐ Colloidal silver
- ☐ Basic makeup essentials and hair accessories
- ☐ Bottle of water

Food Preparation Essentials

Whether you've had a vaginal or cesarean delivery, having meals and snacks prepared in advance is going to be super helpful. After a cesarean, it is even more challenging to prepare food in the kitchen, and you are going to want to make sure that your freezer and pantry are well stocked with healthy options for when you bring your baby home. During the first few weeks after your surgery, your meals and eating schedule will likely be fairly scattered. That's okay! Between visits from friends and family, long drawn-out attempts at breastfeeding and showering, and possibly even toddler naps you may still be dealing with, sticking to your perfect eating schedule right after the baby arrives is pretty much unattainable. LET... IT... GO! I promise you will get there again, but for now, eat when you are hungry and don't worry about every meal being amazing and on time. Having healthy snacks that qualify as meals, such a healthy muffins, soups, fruit and veggies, and homemade energy bars can go a long way in nourishing you and your family while not adding too much extra preparation or cleanup time. On top of having a well-stocked freezer and pantry, I highly recommend having your support partner or a close friend or family member do a last-minute grocery store pickup before your last day at the hospital. This way, you'll also be stocked with fresh fruits and veggies as soon as you walk through the door. And don't hesitate to use disposable dishes for a while too!

Let's talk about the meal train! If you have never heard of this before, it is when friends and family organize daily meal drop-offs for you after you've had a baby. Even if it isn't totally organized, you may be in a position where you have many friends and family bringing you all kinds of casseroles and meals. Often, churches, families, or care groups will set up a meal train in advance for new moms. If this is you, count yourself blessed!

Meal trains are one way others can show you how much they care, and at times they will come in super handy. However, I still highly suggest you have your own favorite meals prepared in advance and stored in the freezer instead of completely relying on other people to bring you your meals.

So many times, we had amazing friends and family offer to bring hot, ready-to-eat dinners to our home. They would offer to drop it off during a certain time frame, and we would patiently wait for them to deliver. Although we were always super thankful, our little kiddos sometimes had a hard time waiting, especially if lunch had been a while ago. Or sometimes, part of the meal still needed to be prepared, or perhaps it was even something that our other kids were not familiar with eating. Depending on your personal eating preferences, there may even be meals with ingredients that can bother you or your new baby's tummy. This is where it's super handy to have other options available to feed both you and your family.

Of course, you can enjoy the meals offered by friends and family, and I am so grateful for the meals we received. I just want to remind you that when you're dealing with a new baby, establishing a milk supply, healing from a surgery, and feeling completely exhausted, it's just not the time to force your family to eat things they are unfamiliar with. I am only suggesting that you don't solely rely on the meal trains for your *entire* menu plan. It is always good to have other options available that you know will fuel your family well. You can always pop these gifted meals into the freezer for another day. Most of them save very well!

What Items are Most Beneficial to Stock in the Freezer or Pantry?

First and foremost, I always make sure I have a good supply of healthier cookies and muffins for the kids, along with some lactation baked goods (homemade cookies, muffins, or granola bars that specifically include ingredients that are known to increase and support your milk supply) available for myself. Having these snacks on hand will also come in handy when the breastfeeding munchies hit full force. (Something about coming out of surgery while starting the lactation process all over again always makes me ravenously hungry!) You don't have to search long and hard to find some amazing recipes for lactation cookies, muffins, and other treats that will be amazing to add into your diet. Feel free to experiment with a few in advance to make sure you find the ones that you'll enjoy the most.

If you're a soup person, I recommend having some of your favorite soups either canned in advance or frozen in the freezer. Depending on the size of your family, you may find it beneficial to save them in smaller, individual size portions, or you may find it easier to freeze an entire meal's worth for the whole family at a time. Some soups that save particularly well are vegetable soups, chicken noodle soups, potato soups, stews, and chili. Just be aware of overdoing on ingredients that could upset your new baby's tummy when digested through your breastmilk.

It's always best to start off with a blander diet and slowly introduce new foods over time to monitor how the baby reacts to your breastmilk. One of my babies was super sensitive to what I ate, while for the most part the others seemed to hardly be affected. I suggest taking the first few weeks while you are catching up from the surgery to restrain from foods that could be a potential trigger, at least while you are healing. Then you won't need to second guess why your baby is fussing based on the foods you ate. It's one less thing to worry about!

Some common foods that have been known to cause babies' tummies to become gassy or upset are dairy products; caffeine-containing foods including soft drinks, chocolate, coffee, and some teas; spicy foods such as strong spices or garlic cloves; and broccoli, onions, Brussels sprouts, green peppers, cauliflower, cabbage, and tomatoes. Although most vegetables are much better when cooked than in their raw state, personal breastfeeding experiences confirm that gassy foods can make gassy babies. I always wait a few weeks until introducing those foods just to be safe!

You'll also want to have several hearty and heavy ready-to-go meals that you will absolutely look forward to eating when you come home. Getting out of your hospital bed and back into your home is such a refreshing feeling, and being able to eat something other than fast food, hospital food, and snacks will also feel SO amazing. Have at least a few meals for the first week ready to go, such as your favorite meat and potatoes, stir fry, or a hearty meal of pasta and sauce. For the most part, these meals also freeze very well and can be made into individual or family-size portions.

Having some caffeine-free teas on hand, especially if you are a tea drinker, is also a good idea. There are many healing herbal teas available that are specifically designed for new moms.

If you have other kids at home, have some of their favorite snacks available too, even the ones that might not be the healthiest option. Bringing a baby home is a big deal for them, too, and sometimes their favorite mini chocolate bars, crackers, or chips, or even popcorn can go a long way in treating them to something special.

Having some packaged options available can be helpful in a pinch. Even though they are not the healthiest option, sometimes you just have to do what you can to get through the day. Boxed pasta, store-bought soup, or even Costco-sized casseroles can be lifesavers at times!

Freezer and Pantry Checklist

- ☐ Muffins, cookies, and energy bars for the kids
- ☐ Lactation cookies for Mom
- ☐ Several different soup options, either in family- or personal-sized portions
- ☐ At least seven hearty meal options for the first week that freeze well
- ☐ A good supply of nourishing and relaxing teas
- ☐ Treats for the kids
- ☐ Easy to make packaged options such as pasta, canned soup, or store-bought casseroles
- ☐ Disposable dishes

The Essentials of Preparing Your Home for Siblings

If this is not your first rodeo as a new mom, you likely have other children in the home waiting for your full attention the exact moment you walk through the door. Although I touch more on this in Chapter 12, I want to specifically dive into the things you can do in the weeks and months leading up to your cesarean that will make life with a new baby easier while not neglecting the other children in the house.

My first suggestion to all moms with littles at home is that if your kids are not already used to having quiet time in the afternoon, start this habit as early on in your pregnancy as you can. Even as my kids grew out of their afternoon naps, we have consistently implemented quiet time in our house, even when I wasn't pregnant. For our family, quiet time simply means an hour or two after lunch is cleaned up when the kids are required to play quietly in their rooms, read or look at books, or quietly watch a show. (The only exception to this rule is that once they are old enough to play independently outside, they are allowed to play outdoors rather than indoors if the weather will cooperate.) When you are recovering from a cesarean or when a new baby is brought home, you'll need this quiet time in the afternoon to rest, breastfeed, and simply clear your head from the new baby confusion. Just as it is super important to get up and move after a cesarean, it is also important to find time to rest. Implement a quiet-time routine for your kids early on, and it will stick with you for years!

Try to have the laundry as caught-up as possible before you go in for your surgery. With other kids at home, it is difficult to ever actually fully "catch up," but you can try to stay on top of the laundry pile. This will be especially helpful if you end up going in earlier than expected, and yes, it happens more often than you think. This is a great time to get hubby or your significant other involved if he hasn't already been helping out.

If you have the type of toddler who likes to try on ten-plus outfits a day (like my first daughter), put their clothes out of reach for a while so they can't pull apart their dresser within the first five minutes of waking up. Even just keeping their clean clothes in a basket out of reach can save you an enormous amount of sorting and organizing. Bending over during the last weeks of pregnancy and the first weeks after a cesarean is not fun, and you should avoid it as much as possible.

De-clutter all of your toys weeks before your cesarean date, leaving only a few special toys out for the kids to play with. You'll be surprised how creative your kids will be with less stuff and how much easier this makes coming home from the hospital. Bending over and picking up toys while healing is not necessary. You also don't want your kids to constantly hear you nagging at them to pick up everything amongst the craziness that already comes with a new baby. When it comes to healing from your cesarean, think "less is more." If you have time leading up to your due date, take the time to buy each child a new special toy and a few activity books they can play with after the baby comes home. This will help keep them busy or quiet as needed and also make them feel like they are special, too.

Preparing Your Home for Siblings Checklist

- ☐ Start a quiet-time routine
- ☐ Stay on top of laundry as much as possible
- ☐ Declutter their clothes and toys
- ☐ Get them each a special surprise for when baby comes home that will help keep them occupied for quiet times

Having your home prepared will seriously make all the difference when you come home after your surgery. You are going to want to focus on healing, rest, and bonding with your new baby rather than making meals, doing dishes, and cleaning up after everyone. Doing a few small things in advance will ensure that you have the best outcome possible.

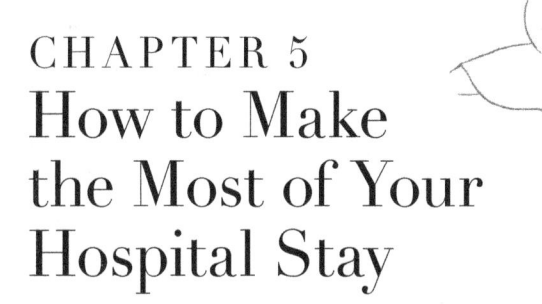

CHAPTER 5
How to Make the Most of Your Hospital Stay

What to pack in your hospital bags for you, your support partner, and your baby to make the most out of your hospital stay.

THE TYPE OF DELIVERY you have will determine how long you can expect to stay at the hospital after your baby is born. A hospital stay after a vaginal delivery is generally one to two nights, whereas the stay after a cesarean is usually about three nights long. Even though that doesn't seem like a very long stay, it is extremely beneficial to be well prepared while you are there. After all, you want both you and your support partner to enjoy this time together as much as possible rather than having him running around looking for all of the things that you forgot!

When I went in for my last cesarean, the hospital was extremely busy and the staff seemed to have very little time to check on me or the baby. With the exception of having our vitals checked, we were pretty much left on our own, which was actually really nice since this was our seventh time around. However, after only twenty-four hours, they asked if we would be okay with an early discharge. I was actually shocked! That is a very short amount of time to have medical care after a cesarean before they send you home. It almost felt like we were filling out the discharge papers before we had even settled in. However, had we not been prepared with the proper clothing, car seat, identification cards, etc., that could easily have been a very stressful situation. But since we were well prepared, we could easily access everything we needed to quickly fill out the papers and make our journey home.

I usually like to have my hospital bags packed and ready to go between weeks thirty and thirty-five. Pending no extreme emergencies, this will definitely give you enough time to prepare while continuing to think things over well before the baby arrives. Packing for the hospital while preparing for a cesarean requires a few extra essential items that you wouldn't have in your bags for a vaginal delivery. Even if you're planning a vaginal delivery, having these extra items on hand can definitely come in handy if things suddenly go in a different direction than you were expecting. Remember, you want to pack light, so just think that everything that goes in also has to come out… including the baby in a car seat. And because you will not be able to lift anything at all, loading the car when it comes time to go home will completely fall on your support partner. It gets even more difficult if the weather is miserable and you can't park close to the front doors of the hospital. I definitely suggest you call ahead to see what your hospital's parking, pickup, and drop-off protocol looks like before heading in for the first time.

It's also common to not be given a room until after your cesarean. In some cases, the hospital may require you to leave your bags in the car (or elsewhere) until you're assigned a room once your surgery is over. Ask your hospital about their specific policies in advance!

Listed below are my go-to, must-haves. I've used these lists over and over again, and I've also included the reasoning behind some of the items in case you aren't sure why they would be so important to have in the hospital. Here we go:

Packing List for Mom

- ☐ **COMFORTABLE SLIPPERS:** Ideally, you will want ones that have grips and are easy to slip on and off. You won't want to bend down to pull them over your heels. Some moms find that their feet swell after surgery too, so it is not a bad idea to size up or at least make sure they have some extra room.

- ☐ **FLIP-FLOPS:** Keeping your balance immediately following a cesarean can be difficult at times. The last thing you'll want to do is to slip in the shower after your surgery. You'll want your flip-flops to have fairly good grips on the bottom too. And even if you are having a vaginal delivery, it is a good idea to bring flip-flops just so you can avoid stepping on the bare floor of the shower. Even though the shower has likely been recently cleaned, it is still not your own. I just can't help being slightly grossed out thinking about all the things that have likely happened in there before me.

- ☐ **NURSING BRA:** Your nursing bra should easily undo to make feeding your baby a bit easier. Even if you choose to go bra-less for part of the day, you'll want something available if you have guests or for when you go home.

- ☐ **NIPPLE CREAM:** A high-quality, natural nipple cream is always a must. Your nipples can take quite the beating at the beginning, and these creams go a long way in preventing them from cracking. As mentioned earlier, this is where colloidal silver gel has become such a life saver for me. It assists with healing quickly, feels amazing, and is completely safe for baby.

- ☐ **NURSING PADS:** These can be either disposable or reusable. I always prefer the disposable option for my hospital stays.

- ☐ **NURSING PILLOW:** Bring along a nursing pillow that helps you elevate your baby while breastfeeding and snuggling. It can be very difficult at first to keep your baby lifted into position, and a nursing pillow helps you remain comfortable while experimenting with different positions without being too strenuous on your body.

- ☐ **NURSING GOWN THAT BUTTONS IN THE FRONT:** Some moms love to wear these as soon as they are able to change. Having something loose around your abdomen and incision can feel refreshing, plus it makes it much easier to access both for breastfeeding and for the nursing staff to monitor your incision.

- ☐ **HIGH-WAISTED COMPRESSION LEGGINGS OR SHORTS:** For me, these have always been my go-to pants of choice in the hospital. I preferred to have something to hold it altogether and add some compression over my incision. Bring more than one pair in case you bleed through your pad, which is actually very common.

- ☐ **NURSING TOPS:** I always bring a good quality tank for sleeping in, and another two nursing tops for at the hospital.

- ☐ **CARDIGAN:** The temperature in the hospital rooms is constantly changing, or at least that's what it feels like. Having a cozy cardigan that you can slip on and off as needed is perfect.

- ☐ **HIGH-WAISTED UNDERWEAR:** You'll be given disposable maternity underwear after your procedure, and they always have a few extra pairs in the bathrooms, as well. For me, this was all that I used. They hold everything in, keep your pads in place, and can be pulled right over your incision for gentle comfort. If you would rather have your own, or in case your hospital does not offer extra pairs, it's a good idea to bring some of your own too.

- ☐ **SOCKS:** Bring a few pairs to keep your feet warm.

- ☐ **ABDOMINAL BAND:** If you can find one specifically for cesareans, they are truly the best thing you can add to your hospital bag, and you should continue wearing it once you return home. If you can't find one specifically for cesareans, any abdominal band that can support your core after your procedure will do wonders in speeding up your recovery and making those first few weeks much more bearable.

- ☐ **A FAMILIAR PILLOW:** The hospital pillows are usually pretty uncomfortable. Bring along your own to help you sleep just a little bit better.

- ☐ **A SMALL THROW BLANKET:** A little blanket that makes it feel a little more like home is so helpful. The hospital blankets can feel quite scratchy, cold, and uncomfortable.

- ☐ **COMFORTABLE SHOES:** You will want something comfortable with grips to go home in.

- ☐ **EXTRA-LARGE WATER BOTTLE:** You are going to be so, SO thirsty after your cesarean. Ideally, bring a water bottle that also keeps things icy cold. You will want a fairly large one as you will be drinking a lot of water!

- ☐ **HAIR ACCESSORIES:** Pack a brush, some hair ties, bobby pins, and whatever else you most commonly use in your hair. Think simple styles, as even lifting your hands above your head can feel draining at first.

- ☐ **LIP GLOSS:** You will want one that is super moisturizing. The air in the hospitals can be very dry, and this will go a long way in keeping your lips from cracking open.

- ☐ **LOTION:** This will help keep your skin moist in the dry room.

- ☐ **TOOTHBRUSH, TOOTHPASTE, AND DEODORANT:** *No need to explain!*

- ☐ **Q-TIPS, TWEEZERS, AND NAIL CLIPPERS:** I have learned in life to never be without these! You always need them when you least expect it.

- ☐ **MAKEUP AND A SMALL MIRROR:** If you are someone who likes to wear a bit of color on your face to feel refreshed, you'll want a few of your favorite items in a small bag that you can keep close to your bed. I always brought a tiny mirror so I could freshen up in my bed without having to walk around the room.

- ☐ **SHAMPOO, CONDITIONER, AND BODY WASH:** You will likely have a shower or two before you go home, so definitely pack along your favorite shampoo and conditioner, as well as some gentle body soap. It feels so amazing to get cleaned up after they have taken your IV and catheter out.

- ☐ **TOWEL AND FACE CLOTH:** I always prefer to bring one of my own, although the hospital will also provide these for you.

- ☐ **VITAMINS AND MEDICATION:** Although most hospitals provide you with prenatal vitamins in your medicine pack, I always preferred using my own. Be sure to bring along whatever your regular vitamin and medication routine is.

- ☐ **PEPPERMINT ESSENTIAL OIL:** You will have a lot of extra abdominal gas left after your procedure. This can often move to your shoulder and cause extreme pain, sometimes lasting for up to a week. I have tried many things to relieve this pain, however the only thing that ever actually gave me relief was peppermint essential oil. Simply mix it with a carrier oil, such as coconut oil, and rub it around your upper abdomen and on your shoulders where you have pain (obviously staying far away from your incision and your breasts).

- ☐ **NURSING TEA:** This can be picked up online or at any health food store. It is a great option to enjoy that will go a long way in supporting your milk supply. More about this later.

- ☐ **CHIA SEEDS:** Chia seeds are something I would never go without at the hospital. They do not need a fridge to be stored short term and are an excellent source to add to your toast, yogurts, or oatmeal the hospital provides. Chia seeds added to your meals will also go such a long way in helping your first bowel movement along. I talk more about these in Chapter 13.

- ☐ **SNACKS:** You will likely get very tired of the hospital food that is provided and will want a few of your favorite snacks tucked away in your purse.

- ☐ **A SLEEP MASK:** If you prefer a dark room when you sleep, you may want to throw one of these in your bag. Some rooms remain fairly bright at night with constant interruptions from the nurses, especially if you are in a shared space. A sleep mask can help a little.

- ☐ **PHONE AND PHONE CHARGER:** *Obviously!*

- ☐ **WALLET:** You'll want to bring your wallet with all of your insurance papers, health cards, identification, etc. You'll likely have several papers to fill out before you leave that require the information on those documents, and you will also want to bring along some money for parking, vending machines, and cafeteria food.

Packing List for Dad or Your Support Partner

- ☐ **AT LEAST TWO SETS OF CLOTHING**: If they are planning on staying overnight, they will want a few changes of clothes, including socks and underwear.
- ☐ **SLEEPWEAR**: Bring along whatever they are most comfortable sleeping in.
- ☐ **FLIP-FLOPS**: If they plan on staying overnight and showering, these will come in handy.
- ☐ **TOILETRIES**: Everything they regularly use such as toothbrush, toothpaste, deodorant, etc.
- ☐ **TOWELS AND FACE CLOTHS**: Bring an extra set if they prefer to use their own.
- ☐ **SNACKS**: The hospital does not provide food for support partners. Make sure you bring some extras along for them, too.
- ☐ **WATER BOTTLE**: One that keeps the water icy cold is ideal.
- ☐ **LIP GLOSS**: Yes, their lips get dry too!
- ☐ **FAMILIAR PILLOW**: Your partner will benefit from one of these, as well.
- ☐ **SMALL THROW BLANKET**: To keep them more comfortable if they are staying for the night.
- ☐ **VITAMINS AND MEDICATION**: Bring along whatever they normally take at home.
- ☐ **PHONE AND PHONE CHARGER**: Obviously!
- ☐ **WALLET**: They may need to assist with filling out the paperwork before you are discharged. They'll also want to bring along some money for parking, vending machines, and cafeteria food.

Packing List for Baby

- ☐ **DIAPERS:** The hospital generally provides these for you; however, it is always a good idea to have a few extra just in case.

- ☐ **WIPES:** Some hospitals provide disposable wipes while others have you use wet cloths or paper towels. I prefer having my own wipes on hand, so that I don't have to climb in and out of bed just to change the baby.

- ☐ **SLEEPERS:** Bring four to five sleepers. It may seem like a lot for just a couple days, but they end up getting dirty more often than you think!

- ☐ **COMING-HOME OUTFIT:** I usually bring along two options in case one gets dirty or we have a change in the weather. Consider the weather in your area when making your choices.

- ☐ **HATS OR TOQUES:** A baby's head tends to get a bit cold once they are introduced to their new world outside of their mama's tummy. Something on their heads will keep them nice and cozy.

- ☐ **COMFORTABLE HEAD BOWS:** If you have a little girl, you might want to bring along some comfortable bows for those first adorable pictures!

- ☐ **BABY MITTENS OR SOCKS:** Newborns' nails are often fairly long and scratchy, and you won't want to fuss with clipping or filing them right away. Having mitts to prevent them from scratching themselves is ideal. I actually preferred to put tiny socks on their hands as they seemed to stay on better than the mittens.

- ☐ **DIAPER CREAM:** A baby's first poops are very sticky. You'll want to always have a layer of cream between their skin and their diaper to make changing them much easier. Most hospitals provide Vaseline, however you may prefer to have a more natural option.

- ☐ **SWADDLING BLANKETS:** You'll want two to three swaddling blankets to keep your baby swaddled up and cozy.

- ☐ **BABY BLANKETS:** I always bring a few extra blankets just to lay them down on the bed when changing the baby or as an extra layer of softness in the hospital bassinet. The ones provided at the hospital are often washed in strong detergent or can be scratchier than you would prefer.

- ☐ **CAR SEAT:** You'll be required to have an up-to-date car seat to take your baby home. In fact, most if not all hospitals require a car seat check before they will allow your baby to be discharged. Make sure it is set up before you head into the hospital and not expired!

- ☐ **CAR SEAT COVER:** A canopy or cover to throw over the car seat will help keep your baby warm and cozy. If it's summer, choose something lighter that keeps the wind and sun out without having them overheat.

CHAPTER 6

Gentle, Natural, and Family-Centered Birth Plan

Understanding the birthing options that may be available to you even if you are undergoing a cesarean delivery.

AS YOU PROBABLY figured out by now, my first cesarean happened in a pretty scary and panicked state, and because I was completely unprepared for the situation, I had absolutely no birth plan, wishes, or suggestions for my surgery. I was completely left alone at the whim of the medical team. And because it was already an emergency situation and they had absolutely no prior relationship with me, we were complete strangers. Without a birth plan, there was no way for them to tell what things were important to me regarding the delivery and aftercare of myself or my baby. Although it is true that in an emergency situation it will be much more difficult for all of your wishes to be followed, there are still some things I could have written down in advance that might have gone a long way in preventing some of the drama I experienced both during and after the cesarean.

One of the first things I can remember—which still gives me anxiety thinking about it to this day—is when they strapped my hands to the side of the operating table. They said it was to help hold me still and prevent me from panicking more. However, had they given me the option at the time, I would have not wiggled a bit if it meant I was able to have my arms free and at least hold my husband's hand or move my hair or my glasses into a better position. How awful and intrusive it was to not only fear that my newborn baby was not going to make it, but then to be strapped to a table as if I were some kind of an animal with zero control. It only made an already very fearful situation worse.

And if that wasn't bad enough, after he was born and proven to be healthy, they passed my little baby to me but refused to let us have skin-to-skin time. Skin to skin (also known as kangaroo care) is simply the act of letting your fresh, unclothed baby lay on your bare chest. Skin-to-skin care has been proven to improve babies' temperature, stabilize their heart rate, decrease crying, improve oxygen saturation, improve breastfeeding outcomes, and so much more. The nurse we had at the time was extremely difficult and told me that the freezing from my spinal tap needed to come out a lot more before I could hold him the way I wanted or attempt to breastfeed him. I kept telling her over and over that I was ready, but she seemed more than eager to deny me this opportunity for what seemed like forever. It was not a good experience at all. I felt that I had lost such an important aspect of bonding with my new son. With the exception of a medical emergency, all moms and dads should have the opportunity to immediately have skin-to-skin time with their newborn baby! It is my hope that sharing my experiences with you will prevent you from encountering a similar situation. While it's true that, depending on your level of freezing, you may want to wait a bit to breastfeed so that you can fully feel the latch, most women feel confident enough to make this decision on their own and not have a nurse decide for them. This is an option you can have in writing in your birth plan to help your medical team understand your needs.

More and more moms and moms-to-be long to take a much more natural and calming approach to their cesareans, and many hospitals are taking note! Usually referred to as a "gentle cesarean," these cesareans make a much greater effort to respect the mom's wishes for her birth so that she is able to replicate, as closely as possible, the birth that she always dreamed of having—even if it ends up as a cesarean. Oh, how I wish I had a birth plan prepared in advance with my first babies! Of course, there are many aspects that you can't replicate in a gentle cesarean, such as a medicated-free birth; however, a mom-to-be actually has many options available to her. Some hospitals are amazing at going the extra distance to accommodate these wishes as best as they safely and medically can; however, other hospitals tend to be much more difficult to work with. Sadly, I have experienced both types of cesareans and it makes an amazing difference when you work with a doctor who tries to respect your wishes as much as possible. Just like a vaginal birth, it's an excellent idea to write, in advance, a simple birth plan, complete with your signature, that has all of your hopes and wishes in the event you end up with a cesarean.

In my experience, I feel that a lot has changed for the better in the last fourteen years when it comes to labor and delivery. Over time, I have found that the cesarean and hospital experience has only improved. My last three babies were delivered by an excellent OB/GYN, who was so careful about asking me about my wishes ahead of time that I didn't even need to have a birth plan in place. Of course, it is still a good idea to have one ready anyway, should you end up going in earlier than expected or if you end up with a doctor on-call rather than the one you've been seeing throughout your pregnancy.

So, What Kinds of Things Can You Actually Request in a Cesarean Birth Plan?

A lot, actually. Because this book is mainly about cesarean delivery, I won't include the items that you may request in the event that you are first attempting a vaginal birth. I will also not include other things you may want to consider, such as the tests and procedures that all hospitals have in their protocols for newborn babies. Again, many books and amazing podcasts and videos have been created that can go a long way in informing you with all of the choices that are available to you and your baby. My goal is to focus on the cesarean advice I so tenderly want to share with you. Birth is a complicated process, and it is good to research all areas involving this important event. However, in this particular book, I only want to include the things helpful in a specific *cesarean* birth plan!

The more I researched, the more control I realized that I had. And trust me, the more you feel in control of several aspects of your cesarean, the calmer you will feel. Below is a list of the things you might want to include on your cesarean birth plan. You don't necessarily need to include all of these as maybe they will not be important to you at the time. Remember, some hospitals will have protocols in place that simply do not allow for all of your wishes to be accommodated, but it doesn't hurt to ask.

- Ask if you can have a clear surgical drape rather than a blue one in place for the actual delivery. This will allow you to see the baby being born. Some hospitals even have mirrors that you can use to better see the baby as it is delivered.

(I personally loved the clear drape, but I never asked for a mirror—just not my cup of tea, I guess!)

- Ask that your hands remain completely free from being strapped down. In most cases, I feel that this is a complete violation of a mother's right in birthing her babies.

- Let your medical team know in advance if you do not want to be operated on by a resident or intern doctor.

- Ask if you can have your IV placed on your non-dominant arm so it is easier to hold and maneuver your baby once they are born.

- Make sure it is okay that your support partner takes videos and pictures during the birth. I have never heard them not allow this, but as always it is a good idea to check.

- If you have a doula or a midwife you are working with during your pregnancy, you should ask if they allow an extra support person in the room. I asked once to have a doula/photographer join me for the delivery, but the hospital's policy was to only allow one support partner. I have, however, talked with women who were allowed to have a doula along with their partner.

- If you want specific music played during the surgery, ask. Many hospitals are more than happy to accommodate this request.

- Feel free to ask the staff to keep their personal conversations to themselves if you would rather have a quiet environment to birth your baby. Or, on the contrary, don't hesitate to ask them to keep on making small talk if you feel it will calm your nerves.

- You may ask to have your husband or support partner cut the cord if this is important to you.

- You have the option of asking for delayed cord clamping if this is important to you. If it is deemed safe at the time, many hospitals will accommodate this request.

- You may request that your husband or care partner announces the sex of your baby rather than the doctor, even if you already know what it is!

- You may ask that you can hold your baby skin to skin as soon as possible. This can also include putting baby on the breast as early as deemed safe. Some hospitals will even allow you to delay the testing and newborn assessments so that you can immediately hold your baby if they feel it is safe to do so.

- You may ask that they do not swaddle or place a hat on your baby if you would rather have them skin to skin immediately.

- You may include the option to drink water as soon as possible after surgery. I have had a few instances where the nurses made me wait a desperately long time, which completely affected my ability to relax and enjoy the baby. I know they want to make sure you are able to "hold things down" before you fill up with fluids, but in most cases, if you are feeling well, you should be able to have access to water.

- Ask to have the IV and catheter removed as soon as possible after surgery. Some nurses are okay to do it sooner if you are moving around and drinking plenty of fluids.

- In the event that your baby needs extra medical attention, ask that your support person is able to stay with your baby as much as possible and be involved with the medical decisions being made and/or discussed.

The first time I had a baby taken to the NICU, the pediatrician involved was cold and harsh with both me and my husband, and she had absolutely no respect for us even though we were completely frightened. She basically whisked the baby away behind a curtain and whispered among herself and the nurses as to what was going on while they monitored his vitals more closely. Every time my husband or I asked for more details, she was rude and acted as though we had no right to know. This again is a complete violation of the parents' rights. You have every right to know the details of what is happening to your baby. Even if it is such an intense emergency that the baby needs to be rushed away, you can still ask to be treated with respect and given all of the details accurately as soon as it is medically possible.

I wish so badly that each and every mom who is reading this book could have every single one of her wishes granted during her labor and delivery—regardless of whether it is a vaginal or cesarean birth. But, as with anything in life, part of the journey is accepting and growing from the little surprises and unknowns that are thrown our way. The way you approach your medical team will also go a long way in keeping the birth experience positive. Even if your nurses or doctors don't agree with you or seem to view things differently than you do, most are still eager to listen and accommodate, especially when spoken to with respect. Remember, in the end, what everyone wants is the most positive outcome for you and your baby. You can still be firm in your beliefs while remaining respectful to all of the others involved. Always approach each situation with a listening ear and open mind, and don't hesitate to ask for more information before proceeding with any major decisions.

In the end, what matters most is that you and your baby are healthy. Enjoy the process from start to finish, remembering that every event that happens in your life can either be used for good or for bad. Even the most stressful and unplanned moments in life can be used to strengthen yourself and others if you handle them with care. Don't let your suddenly interrupted plans allow you to become angry and bitter or to feel worthless. Rather, use them to inspire yourself to push for growth and become the best mom and person, even amongst all of the little challenges that life continues to throw your way.

CHAPTER 7

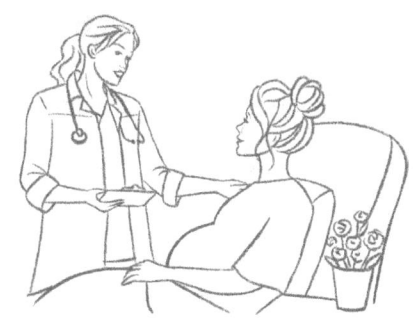

The Day Has Arrived

What to expect the morning of your
cesarean and the first few hours
after arriving at the hospital.

THE DAY OF your scheduled cesarean is finally here. First of all, I want to give you a huge congratulations! Carrying a baby is no easy task. You are probably filled with a ton of emotions today: excited about meeting your precious baby; nervous about the delivery; energized because this day has finally arrived; exhausted because you are at the end of a long pregnancy; sad that you are done carrying this little one in your tummy; and scared because you are not entirely sure what to expect. And lastly and most understandably, completely overwhelmed. It all feels so surreal. In a few hours you are going to be holding your new little baby and saying goodbye to one stage of your life and entering into another. Know that ALL of these emotions are normal, healthy, and a complete testament to the amazing mom and strong woman that you are!

Preparation at Home

By now you should already have your hospital bag, your partner's hospital bag, and your baby's hospital bag ready to go. Have your partner load them into the vehicle while you relax, breathe, and slowly prepare for your cesarean. You aren't allowed to eat anything for the eight hours leading up to your surgery, so you may be starting to feel a little hungry by now. Or perhaps you will find yourself like me where you are so full of butterflies that you have absolutely no appetite anyways. You will, however, be allowed to drink clear liquids for up to two hours before your procedure, so having some calming tea or water is an excellent option. I also always found it super helpful to have a water bottle full of ice to chew on leading up to the procedure. Not only did this keep me hydrated, but I also found that chewing on ice helped relieve some of the built-up anxiousness I was feeling about the delivery.

Depending on how your hospital prepares for planned cesareans, you may have already received an antibacterial scrub package to use in the shower at home on the morning of your surgery. This would have been given to you at your pre-assessment clinic appointment the week prior to your scheduled cesarean. My last cesarean was in the middle of the covid pandemic, so my pre-assessment clinic happened over the phone. This meant that I was expected to shower at home with my own antibacterial wash before surgery and then again at the hospital once I arrived and was admitted to my room. Your own experience will depend on the care and procedures of your hospital at the time of your cesarean. They will want you to thoroughly scrub down with the antibacterial wash, paying extra attention to your abdomen and upper thighs. The reason they request this is to try to keep you and your environment as sterile as possible to avoid any infection.

The most common type of cesarean incision is a horizontal incision just above your bikini line that is approximately twelve to seventeen centimeters in length, just large enough for your baby's head and body to fit through. The other type of incision is a vertical incision that runs between your naval to your pubic bone. Regardless of which incision your surgeon is planning to make, you will be required to have your pubic hair removed in the area where they make the incision. A nurse at the hospital will either do this for you once you are lying on the operating table and frozen, or you can choose to take care of it at home ahead of time. I always chose to do it at home the morning or the night before; however, the choice is completely up to you.

After your shower at home, I strongly recommend blow-drying your hair or taking the time to braid it or style it in such a way that it will last for a few days, so it'll be easy to maintain after you have your baby. It is quite difficult to move around after your surgery and having your hair more manageable is just one simple step you can do to make your life a little easier over the next few days.

You're not allowed to wear nail polish or heavy makeup during your surgery, but most hospitals allow light makeup. Ask your doctor ahead of time what their requirements are. Because my hospital was okay with a small amount of makeup, I always found it refreshing to apply some mascara, blush, and lip gloss on the morning of the surgery. This is obviously completely based on your personal preference.

Another thing I always found helpful and peaceful was listening to calming music on the drive to the hospital rather than the local news or scrolling on my phone. As small of a detail as this is, I found it important to fill my mind with positivity rather than the hustle and bustle of the current world around me. You'll have plenty of time in the hospital to catch up on news; now is not the time! Let this time be about you, your partner, and your new baby.

Arriving at the Hospital

You'll be asked to arrive at the hospital two hours prior to your scheduled surgery time. This is to ensure the medical staff has enough time to take your blood if needed, wait for the results, start an IV, check your vitals, introduce you to your anesthesiologist, and potentially monitor the baby. You'll also be required to change into a hospital gown, footies, and a cap during this time. Your partner will also be given shoe covers, pants, and a gown; a face mask; and a hair cover ahead of time to put on before he enters the operating room. Your doctor or surgeon will also go over your medical history and walk you through the procedure and answer any questions that you may have. Finally, they'll have you sign a consent form.

Once it gets close to your scheduled cesarean time, you'll be given a sodium bicarbonate antacid drink from one of your nurses—*more about this later.* Trust me, the two hours fly by and, before you know it, you will be holding your baby in your arms! My best advice during this time is to ask as many questions as you have, even if they have already been answered earlier by another nurse or doctor. Sometimes, just talking through your fears out loud is enough to calm your anxiety. It's also good to make small talk with your medical team to lighten the mood a little. I have never had a bad experience during this time and found all of the medical staff to be lighthearted, gentle, knowledgeable, and very caring towards addressing all of my concerns.

Why Would They Need to Take My Blood?

Your doctor might decide to order some specific blood tests before you begin your C-section, depending on your medical history. The tests will provide information about your blood type, blood sugars, and your personal hemoglobin levels. These details will be helpful to your health-care team in the unlikely event that you need a blood transfusion during the C-section.

When I went in for my sixth cesarean, I felt fairly confident in my expectations going into the hospital again. After all, this was definitely not my first rodeo. I had no idea, however, that my doctor was planning on an additional blood test upon arrival to check my hemoglobin levels, and I was completely caught off guard when the nurse mentioned the words *possible blood transfusion!* Even though I had started off the day feeling fairly calm and collected, this one simple test that I was not at all prepared for totally shook me to the core. The thought of needing a blood transfusion completely freaked me out because it was never mentioned in my previous cesareans! I found it much more difficult to calm down prior to the surgery and had really wished I was more prepared for the additional blood work. When you have all of the facts, it's much easier to stay relaxed. Ask your doctor in advance if they plan do any additional blood tests the morning of your C-section so you'll be ready for anything they throw your way!

Although listening to them go over the possibility of a blood transfusion can be and *was* very frightening, the likelihood of one actually happening is very small. Remember, this is just an extra step they are taking to ensure the absolute best care for you and your baby. All other required blood work will be on your prenatal records and will have been gathered earlier in your prenatal appointments.

> **Quick Tip:** Woman who are anemic are two times as likely to require a blood transfusion during or after delivery. Taking an additional iron supplement and eating iron-rich foods can greatly reduce your risk!

Why Do I Need an IV During My C-section?

An IV (intravenous) needs to be started so that the medical team can administer fluids, pain medication, and antibiotics. Once placed, the IV will stay in place for one to two days after your surgery to ensure you stay hydrated until you are eating and drinking enough fluids.

I always hated getting an IV. To be completely honest, this was always my least favorite part, and it's not even because of the pinch. (They really do not hurt that much at all. I promise.) I just get really grossed out at the idea of a needle being placed inside my veins for an extended amount of time. Once in, however, the IV is not really painful either; it's just uncomfortable. Having an IV in my hand made me really struggle with simple tasks like scratching my face (more on this later), eating, drinking, sleeping, and most of all, breastfeeding! Some people have absolutely no issues with IVs, while other people seem to really struggle with them.

> **Quick Tip:** If you think an IV is something that might bother you, definitely consider asking your nurse if they can place it in your non-dominant hand as opposed to your dominant hand. Most of the time they are willing to do it where you request. You'll find it so much easier to hold and feed your baby if your IV isn't in the way on your most commonly used hand.

Why Might They Need to Monitor the Baby in Utero?

This is just another step towards monitoring the health of your baby. Although the pain medication and spinal tap they offer is considered safe for your baby, they may want to make sure your baby's heart is strong and stable before beginning surgery. And moms, please take the time to soak in that precious heartbeat! Even though you'll soon be introduced to your little one on the outside, this will be the last time you'll ever hear them from the inside; it is such a beautiful sound! *Cherish. Every. Last. Minute!*

Why Do I Need to Meet My Anesthesiologist Before the Surgery?

I think for most women, the most dreaded and scary part of the entire surgery is the spinal tap or epidural that is given before the procedure, especially if you have never been frozen or numbed before. Let's face it, the idea of being completely (although temporarily) paralyzed from the abdomen down is kind of intimidating! Not to mention that you will be completely awake and of "sound mind" while they slice through your skin, muscles, and uterus. GROSS! Just the thought of it all can make you nauseous and weak. The anesthesiologist will be able to walk you through the entire process ahead of time, answer your questions, reassure you, and calm your nerves and anxiety. With every single one of my cesareans, the anesthesiologist was always one of the most calming and friendly faces in the operating room. They never hesitated to answer any of my ridiculous questions, always made me feel safe, and validated my concerns.

Why Do I Need an Antacid Drink before Surgery?

This is just to calm down the acid in your stomach in the event that you vomit during surgery. This has never happened to me with any of my cesareans, and chances are you won't experience it either, but being prepared never hurts. Getting acid into your lungs can be dangerous, and this is just an extra safety precaution that is taken. Although the drink does not taste anything like your favorite drink of choice, it's really not that bad; it has more of a salty, bland, odd flavor. Just chug it down and move on!

What Can I Do to Calm Down My Partner?

So, your partner can't seem to keep it together and might be making you more anxious rather than acting as a support person... Yes, I am totally speaking from experience on this one. I know that for many of you, your support person will be a complete rock—encouraging, calming, and reassuring. Although my husband always improves as the day moves on, this was not the case for most of the prep time! More often than not, the minute we would arrive at the hospital his nerves would get the better of him, and he would begin pacing back and forth and making repeated trips to the bathroom. I would be sitting on a bed or in a chair chatting with my medical team and getting prepared for my surgery while he was in and out of the washrooms trying everything in his power to keep it together while feeling like he was failing miserably! It was definitely not calming for me at all. Poor guy!

I'm not sure which side of the fence your support person will fall on; however, I do know that even though they are not the ones on the delivery table, it's still an emotional and anxious thing to go through. Sure, they are not the ones getting cut open, but they are in the operating room, nonetheless, watching someone they love go through something difficult. As much as you need to be supported, remember that they will also need support! Don't forget to reassure them as well and include them in your conversations you have with the medical team. This will go a long way to ensuring you have the best possible experience!

Why Do I Need to Sign a Consent Form?

Signing a consent form is a standard procedure with any surgery. Even though reading through the risks can feel quite intimidating, know that all of the events mentioned are extremely rare and your medical team is more than prepared to handle all of the "what ifs." They are trained to handle any surprises, and the likelihood of anything happening is very, very small. Remember you are in good and qualified hands.

So now that you are ready to go, it is time to sit back, relax, breathe, and take in this time to enjoy how far you have already made it. You are finally in the home stretch! You are prepared, strong, and ready to meet your baby! Good work, Mama!

What if my Cesarean Was Not Planned, and It Ends Up as an Unplanned or Emergency C-section?

Having an unplanned or emergency cesarean when you were not planning or hoping for one can be very difficult to process in the moment. Although having an unplanned or emergency cesarean both end up with the same outcome, there are actually a few differences between the two.

During an unplanned cesarean, the doctor will have had time to discuss the options with the mother if labor and delivery are not progressing as originally planned. Your medical team will likely have time to explain the procedure as they are preparing you for surgery, and the overall situation between everyone involved is often a bit calmer than in an emergency situation. However, just because it is a bit calmer does not mean it is any less heartbreaking to hear. For many moms, this can be a completely devastating moment when they agree to move forward with a cesarean when it goes against everything that they were hoping and praying for. Through your tears and disappointment (which are totally okay and actually part of the healing process), try and keep your eyes and your heart towards your beautiful treasure that you are so close to meeting. I promise everything will be okay—*this is just a new part of your story!*

Unfortunately, during an emergency cesarean, there is often little to no time at all to move forward with the surgery or discuss options, as either the mom, the baby, or both of your lives may be in danger. If this is your case, it is totally normal to be completely scared and overwhelmed. I know I was. Depending on the reason for the emergency cesarean and what state you are in, your doctor will either top up your epidural, administer a spinal tap, or perhaps even put you under general anesthesia. Regardless of what they need to do to get your baby out safely, remember that they are completely prepared and thoroughly trained to handle these situations, and their number-one goal is to get your baby out quickly and safely. As scary as it may be, try and remain calm and let your support partner step in and reassure you as best as they can. *Soon you will be holding your precious baby in your arms!*

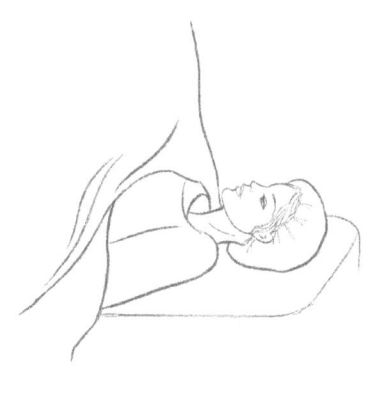

CHAPTER 8
It's GO TIME!

What actually happens during surgery and in the recovery room afterwards?

AHH! IT'S TIME TO GO! You are dressed, your blood work results are in, mom and baby are healthy, and you are on your way! A nurse will now take you *away from your support partner* and head towards the operating room. You are getting SO close!

Wait! What? Why Am I Leaving My Support Partner?

Unfortunately (although probably for the better), your support person is not permitted to enter the operating room until you are completely ready for surgery. While they wait for you, they'll put on their gown and then proceed to wait outside the surgery door until you're ready to go; this usually takes around fifteen to twenty minutes. Don't worry, you are in good hands. Many of the faces you see in the operating room will be people that you've already met in the hours preceding the surgery.

One bonus to having a planned cesarean rather than an emergency cesarean is the casual environment in the operating room. Because there is no immediate rush, all of the staff is relaxed and usually joking around or happily visiting with one another. Use this time and these friendly faces to help you remain calm.

When you enter the surgery room, don't be alarmed with how cold it is! This is to ensure the environment remains sterile. And on the plus side, as soon as your cesarean is complete, you will more than likely be given warm blankets to heat you back up; they feel amazing!

The very first thing they will do once you enter the operating room is have you sit up on the operating table with your gown open to the back so they can administer your freezing medication (most likely a spinal tap). I know you are probably squeamish just from reading this section, but I promise you that it sounds much worse than it feels, and it's honestly not as painful as you are likely imagining. I always use this time to take some deep breaths while I envision holding my baby in my arms. I focus on relaxing my entire body and following the instructions from the anesthesiologist.

Unfortunately, no matter what you do, you can't rush this part. I'm going to say that again because it is REALLY IMPORTANT! *No matter what you do, you cannot rush this part!* As much as you might be dreading this part of the surgery, it has to get done. The more relaxed and calm you are, the faster the anesthesiologist will be able to complete the numbing. Being tense and unsettled just prolongs it. Listen to your anesthesiologist and nurse and make small talk if you need to get your mind onto something else. I have yet to meet an unkind anesthesiologist; in fact, most of them were quite humorous and more than willing to calm my nerves. In all but one of my cesareans, I was offered a pillow to lean into that was held between my body and the nurse in front of me. This helped me to relax, and I would suggest asking for one in advance. If they are able to, I'm sure they'll be more than happy to accommodate this request.

What is a Spinal Tap?

The most common form of numbing or freezing for a planned cesarean is called a spinal tap. In its most simple explanation, a spinal tap is an injection of local anesthetic or numbing medicine that goes directly into your spinal fluid. This will temporarily block your senses from the injection site down to your toes. After it takes effect, almost immediately, you will be completely numb and unable to feel pain or move during the procedure. You'll feel pressure and tugging, but I promise you this does not hurt at all. You will, however, be able to move freely and feel everything above the injection site. Your freezing will typically wear off within two to four hours, depending on the dosage that was used. Slowly, you will begin to feel your toes, and then it will continue upwards until you completely regain full function of your feet, legs, thighs, and abdomen. You will notice some tingling and possibly even itchiness as the freezing wears off; this is completely normal.

What is Epidural Anesthesia?

If a mom-to-be has been in labor for a while and has already received an epidural, this can often be topped up in the event that they go in for an emergency cesarean, as opposed to using a spinal tap. With an epidural, a thin plastic tube or catheter is placed into your spine near the nerves that carry pain messages to your brain. The catheter stays in place in your spine until pain medication is no longer needed, so that it can continue to be topped up as needed. A larger dose of local anesthetic is necessary for an epidural than with a spinal tap, and it takes longer

Your epidural can be topped up if needed whereas a ⟩ cannot. Although an epidural can offer continuous pain relief if needed, it is not as commonly used with cesareans and is a more common option for pain relief during regular labor. Because cesarean procedures generally take less than an hour (in most cases), it isn't necessary to have a continual line for pain relief.

What is General Anesthesia?

Although very unlikely, in some cases general anesthesia may be used. This type of anesthesia will completely put the mom to sleep during delivery. It is only used in an extreme emergency or if the mother has other complications where it is to both her and the baby's benefit to be put under.

The type of anesthesia that will be best for you should be discussed in advance with your doctor and eventually with your anesthesiologist once you arrive at the hospital. They will be able to give you a clear picture of what they recommend as being the best scenario for your situation.

How Common Are Side Effects of Anesthesia?

Although they can happen, side effects from anesthesia are extremely rare. The most common risk factors are pain at the incision site, trouble breathing, itchy skin as the freezing comes out, and least commonly, meningitis. The risk of a meningitis infection is estimated at lower than one in 25,000 to 50,000 cases, and of those cases, many of them were known to have pre-existing conditions that were not particularly clear. Anesthesiologists are very good at what they do! Of all the places your mind can wander during the celebration of your new baby, don't let it go there.

Some women also report feeling like they are not able to breathe properly during the procedure—including me. This is another completely normal part of the surgery. This is because the nerves around the rib cage also become numb, which makes it difficult to feel as though you are actually breathing although, in fact, you are completely fine. The anesthesiologist will be watching your oxygen levels closely and will reassure you during the entire procedure. Don't hesitate to share your concerns with them during the entire process.

I have not personally ever experienced pain after the procedure at the injection site (and I have had seven). However, I have spoken with some other women who have. In most cases, it's just slightly tender and will fade away over time. In very rare cases, some women will continue to have pain for longer periods. In the rare case that this happens to you, know that there are many things you can do to improve this pain and eventually completely heal from this side effect. Your doctor will be able to offer some great suggestions if you find yourself in this situation.

Another common side effect from your spinal tap is the *post-anesthesia itch!* In all seven of my cesareans, I have had this intense itch all over my chest and face as the freezing comes out. Apparently, it is an extremely common—although short-lived—side effect of having a spinal tap. It's the craziest feeling! It felt like I wanted to scratch my face off. It doesn't create a rash or anything, so you don't need to worry about that, and it does go away within a few hours after the surgery. If it is really bad, your nurse can offer you Benadryl to help with the itching. I have had this for some and was able to do without for others. This is up to you!

Let's Move On!

Now that you understand what the different types of anesthesia are along with some of the side effects, let's move on to the rest of the procedure. Because more than likely you'll receive a spinal anesthesia, we are going to focus on that one. If you are having an epidural, they may require you to lie in a different position while they administer it, or you may have already had one that they simply need to top up because you are coming out of a longer labor.

As mentioned already, upon entering the operating room your nurse will have you sit on the operating table. You will already have met most of the people in the operating room, and those that you have not will introduce themselves when you arrive. You'll have your gown on with the open side on your back. You will be asked to sit with your back towards the anesthesiologist and your front will be facing your nurse. Again, If you have the option of using a pillow, I definitely recommend it. It really seemed to help with keeping my back arched and my body relaxed. Your gown will be open (in the back) and your butt will be exposed. This might feel strange to you but trust me, they have seen it all. Nothing new here! They will have you arch your back like a cat as much as you possibly can because they want your spine protruding outwards as much as possible, so they can have a clear view of where to place the needles.

They might ask you if you prefer for them to explain everything as they are doing it or if you'd rather they just go on and get it done without talking about the procedure at all. This is a completely personal preference. Personally, I just wanted to get it done. I did not like discussing what was happening, and I preferred to just lean into the pillow they offered me and breathe my way into my happy place. This is totally up to you! I know other people who are completely opposite to me and would have used a mirror to watch had they been given the opportunity. Everyone is different.

What Do You Mean Needles?
I Thought There Was Only One!

Yes, they actually use more than one needle at the injection site, but this is a good thing... really! First, they will use a local anesthetic to freeze the area where they plan to put in the medicine. Then, they will use a smaller needle to freeze the area a little deeper. After that, they will make several injections until the anesthesia is working properly and you are unable to feel anything from the chest down. Other than pressure, you really don't feel anything at all at this point. It might seem like an eternity, but once it is over, it's all downhill from here—I promise! You are mentally through the toughest point. Breathe. Breathe. Breathe, and think calm and happy thoughts about your baby!

Once the freezing has fully been administered, they will help you slowly lie down on the operating table. Almost instantly you will notice your feet, legs, and abdomen become weightless and numb—and after nine months of carrying this little baby inside, it will actually be a relief to be rid of the strain that a pregnancy puts on your body. This is the part I mentioned earlier in the book where with my first cesarean birth they actually tied my hands down to the operating table to attempt to calm me down. That was probably one of the worst things I have ever experienced with any of my births. It was AWFUL! I highly recommend and strongly encourage you and your partner to advocate to have your hands free. It will create a much more calming experience. It will allow you to hold your partner's hands more easily, scratch your nose, move your glasses around, or just wipe away a tear! You have the right to keep your hands free. Insist on it if you can!

They will now lift up a blue curtain by your chest so that you can't see the majority of the surgery. They'll shave your pubic area if needed, sanitize your belly, and place a catheter to help you urinate, which will remain in place for approximately twelve to twenty-four hours—depending on the hospital's protocols. The only thing you'll be able to feel through all of this is a little tugging. For my last three cesareans, I also had the option of having a clear drape behind the blue curtain so when it came time to deliver the baby, they could drop the blue curtain, and I could watch the baby being delivered. I absolutely love that this has become an option for mothers and think it is such a beautiful way to bring forth your baby, even though you are delivering via cesarean. Seeing my baby delivered through my abdomen did not make me feel squeamish at all. I felt even more connected with those births than any of the previous ones. I would definitely ask if your hospital offers this option.

It will be somewhere during this time that they call your partner into the room. *Finally!* This is when it all starts to get very real. Something about having my husband coming in and holding my hand made everything seem much calmer and more peaceful, and it will likely be the same for you! Make sure he brings a camera or a phone with him to capture all of those beautiful, first few moments; you will be thankful later.

Your anesthesiologist will use an ice cube to test your freezing levels by placing it on various areas of your body to make sure you are completely numb and unable to feel pain during the procedure. Once you are comfortable and lying down with your husband beside you, the medical team will once again go over your details and confirm they are ready to begin. Your care nurse and anesthesiologist will continue monitoring your vitals while visiting with you and your husband. If you want it to be quieter, just ask, or if you want to play music on your husband's phone, you can ask for that too. With my third cesarean, my anesthesiologist actually played music from his phone. It wasn't really my style of music, but it definitely helped to lighten things up a little. If you are feeling nauseous, nervous, cold, or shaky, let your nurse know. These are all normal sensations to feel, and they go away very quickly after your baby arrives.

During your cesarean, your surgeon will need to make both an abdominal incision as well as a uterine incision. As mentioned earlier, the abdominal incision is usually a horizontal incision just above your pubic bone. Once that incision is made, they will then need to make another horizontal incision on the lower portion of your uterus, most commonly known as a low transverse incision. Depending on your situation, other types of incisions on the uterus can also be made if you are experiencing any complications such as placenta previa or extensive scar tissue. (It may seem like forever at the time, but the doctor will let you know very quickly that it is baby time within about ten to twenty minutes after beginning, and this is when they'll drop the blue portion of the curtain (if requested). *The more cesareans you have, the longer this part can take because you may have additional scar tissue they need to cut through.*)

You will likely feel a lot of pressure on your abdomen as they make the incision and move things around internally to prepare your baby for their arrival. It might feel a bit strange, but you will not experience any pain at all. Within seconds of feeling this pressure, the doctor will pull out your baby and clear the baby's mouth and nose of fluids. You'll hear the entire team cheering with excitement and offering up a big congratulations, and most likely even your baby's first cry! Depending on your preferences, they will either clamp and cut the umbilical cord immediately or, if requested, delay this process a little longer while the baby rests on your legs, abdomen, or in the doctor's arms for a few moments. Either your partner or your doctor will announce the sex of the baby and then, depending on your specific scenario, they will likely lay the baby close to your chest for a while so you can get a really close look at and first introduction to your newest little family member. Congratulations, Mama, you made it! Look at the beautiful little baby you made—soak it ALL in.

The moments that follow the arrival of your new little one is where your birth plan can have a major impact on the steps that happen next—pending a healthy birth for both mama and baby.

Babies born during a planned cesarean can sometimes be a little less active at first since their birth was much more of a surprise than if they had to work through hours of contractions prior to being delivered. They may also cry a little less at first and are sometimes a bit sleepier because of the anesthesia that was used earlier. However, babies born via cesarean will generally avoid the "tight squeeze" that accompanies a vaginal birth, and therefore will look a little different than if they had been born vaginally. They are more likely to avoid swelling of their faces, bruising on their cheeks, and temporary flat noses that often accompany a vaginal delivery. And although not always the case, they are slightly more likely to have fluid in their lungs as opposed to a vaginal birth because it was never removed naturally when they squeezed through the birth canal. Your doctor will monitor this just to be sure that they are able to breath okay on their own. In most cases, this generally clears up within a few days and is nothing serious to worry about. Regardless of how they present themselves during those first few moments, you are going to be completely mesmerized by your newest little treasure.

Unless discussed otherwise, the medical crew will quickly wipe the baby down and check out all vitals to make sure your baby is doing well. If everything looks good, they will then pass the baby to your partner to hold. It actually happens quite quickly. While you are falling madly in love with your new little baby, the doctor will stitch both your uterus and abdomen back up. Again you will not feel any pain because of the anesthesia that will still be working at full strength. This can take twenty minutes or more, again depending on your scar tissue, fat tissue, and other factors. However, I promise you will hardly be thinking about them working on you because you'll be so wrapped up with the celebration of your new baby! If you are up to it, you can also hold your baby at this time. They'll ensure your partner is close by in case you feel lightheaded or overwhelmed and want to pass the baby back.

After surgery is complete, they'll take you, your partner, and your baby out to the recovery room. You'll be wrapped up in warm blankets and have special inflating boots placed on your legs to keep your blood flowing. These are very similar to a blood pressure cuff except that they continually inflate and deflate around your lower legs to maintain a healthy blood flow. It can take several hours before you are able to completely feel your feet, legs, and abdomen again from the anesthesia that they administered; however, you will have everything else completely mobile and be more than able to hold and swoon over your baby as long as you are feeling up to it. The exact amount of time it takes for the freezing to wear off can differ for each individual.

During this time, they will monitor your temperature, check your blood flow from your vagina, monitor your incision, and check your freezing with an ice cube. As soon as you feel comfortable, you will be able to put your baby on your breast. Until this time, you will be able to do skin to skin with your baby while you wait. This is where the support partner can also do wonders by bringing you ice chips, holding the baby, making you comfortable, and possibly even calling friends and family to announce your new bundle. I am sure all of your people can't wait to hear the good news!

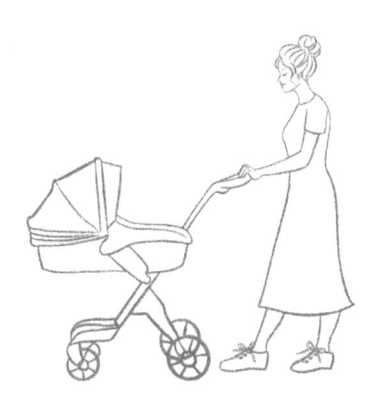

CHAPTER 9
Timeline for Healing from Your Cesarean

How long until I feel like myself again?

AT THE TIME we brought our first baby boy home from the hospital (which seems like an eternity ago), my husband had a temporary position on a dairy farm, and we were living in a quaint, just-under-600-square-feet, cozy apartment in the upper level of a barn shop. Our bedroom window actually faced directly into the shop where our main view was looking at tractors, farm equipment, and pickup trucks. The tiny apartment often smelled liked a mix of diesel fumes and gas, or when we were really *lucky*, those smells might be drowned out by the sewer smell that presented itself every time we turned on the shower or sink. Luxury at its finest! To access the apartment, you had to climb a very long series of wooden steps from the bottom of the concrete floor up to the top of the barn where a small landing led you to our front door. Needless to say, even though we only lived there for a few months, the living accommodations they provided were more than *unique*—definitely not the perfect scenario for bringing home a new baby or healing from a cesarean!

Because we lived about six hours away from all of our friends and family at the time, we were completely flooded with an array of visitors as soon as we came home from the hospital. After all, this was the first grandson for my parents, and the very first grand-baby for my in-laws. It was definitely an exciting arrival. Between my parents, my in-laws, my sisters, and friends, our tiny home was always full of company and adventure. About one week after the baby was born, and soon after my mom had left, my sister-in-law (who was five months pregnant at the time) and her husband came over to meet their new nephew. While we were all inside visiting and doting on my new son, we noticed from the living room window that something was not right outside. As we looked a little closer, we noticed that all of the cows had escaped from the barn and were wandering all over the yard. The owner of the property was away for the day, and we knew that those cows needed to get in the barn promptly!

My husband and brother-in-law raced down the long flight of stairs to begin chasing all of the cows back into the barn. Because I had just had my cesarean and my sister-in-law was pregnant, neither of us were in any position to go down and help them re-capture these dairy cows. Rather, we sat inside on the sofa and watched the drama unfold from inside the cozy apartment. As we watched in suspense, I noticed that the new, young bull had also escaped, and my husband had failed to inform my brother-in-law (who had absolutely zero farm experience) that this little bull was super fiery and something to be extremely wary of!

Within a few moments, we fearfully witnessed the bull approaching closer and closer towards my brother-in-law and then begin bucking and grunting, gearing up to charge him at full force. My brother-in-law was too busy chasing the cows to notice that he was about to be trampled by the bull. I had to act immediately. Without much of a thought, I flew down the long wooden steps and out of the front door as quickly as I could and continued to scream out to my brother-in-law to jump out of the way! Luckily, he jumped just in time and landed in some snow-covered farm equipment and the bull dodged into another direction right at the last moment.

Although I was glad that he was safe, my quick series of reactions was the worst thing I could have done with a fairly fresh incision. Unfortunately, I managed to completely rip my cesarean open, and it became severely infected. Within a few days, I ended up back in the hospital and needed intravenous antibiotics administered to combat the infection while they stitched my cesarean back up again. It was painful, exhausting with a newborn, and frankly quite terrifying. What should have been a six-week recovery period after my baby was born turned into a much more dramatic recovery than anything I had prepared for. Although the hospital had sent me home with a few pamphlets and papers that list the typical timeline for healing, recovering from a major abdominal surgery can look very different for each individual depending on their unique situation—like it did for me!

I'll detail the most common timeline for healing from your cesarean and what you can generally expect after having your baby. Although my first cesarean was a dreadful recovery process, my next six births were much more predictable. However, you need to remember that each body and situation is unique. Some moms have a lot of extra support at home, while others are going to be expected to do a lot more on their own. Some moms are having their first baby, while others are coming home to a house full of toddlers or older children. The best thing you can do is listen to your body and take each moment as it comes. Try not to rush or push yourself more than you are ready for at the time. Our bodies are very capable of healing themselves properly if we give them the precious time and tools that they require.

Initial Hour After Surgery

As mentioned earlier, immediately following your surgery, both you and your baby will be moved to a post-operative recovery area where you'll by monitored by a nurse. Your support partner will be able to stay with you the entire time. A nurse will likely give you warming blankets to raise your temperature. (They feel amazing after coming out of the cold, surgical room). They will also apply the inflatable boots I mentioned earlier on your legs to help keep your blood flowing well around your body. Although the boots feel a little silly and make a bit of noise, you won't notice them right away until the freezing starts to wear off. Basically, they are just casts that wrap around your legs and fasten with Velcro. They feel similar to a blood pressure cuff. Most hospitals will expect you to wear these for the first day or so, or at least until you are up and moving on your own. You get used to them pretty quickly. They are also easy to adjust on your own once you are able to sit and move more freely if they start to feel loose or tight.

The recovery nurse will check for things like bleeding from your vagina and incision area, as well as continue to take your temperature and blood pressure. Remember, just because you have a cesarean does not mean that you do not bleed from your vagina too. (This actually came as quite a shock to me at first as I assumed that they naturally "cleaned" everything out when they took out the baby.) They will also be constantly checking to see how your freezing is wearing off and asking you questions about your pain. At this point, you will still have a catheter in for your urine, so you do not need to get up to use the washroom, as well as an IV to administer fluids. As long as you don't have any complications, you will be able to hold your baby and begin skin-to-skin contact, as well as begin breastfeeding right away.

The Remainder of Day One

After you've been cleared from the post-operative recovery area, you, your support partner, and your baby will move to your room, where you'll stay for the remainder of your time at the hospital. A nurse will continue to check on you often. Because of the anesthesia and pain medication, you'll likely still not be feeling any pain at this time. The pain medication they administered via your IV earlier will generally wear off within eighteen hours. Your nurse will start by offering you ice chips and small sips of water while they continue to monitor you closely. Once they confirm you can handle the ice chips and water, you'll be offered a piece of toast or a light meal, usually within eight hours of your surgery, or sometimes even sooner. By this time, you might be getting fairly hungry! From here, you will be able to continue bonding with your new baby and hopefully get some rest. It's surprising how tired you'll feel after the entire ordeal is over.

Within about six to twelve hours after your surgery, they are going to want you to get up and walk. The first time they came into my room to ask me to get up, I thought, *Are you crazy!* I had just had a major abdominal surgery, and I felt in no way ready to get up and move. However, with the help of your nurse, who will organize your IV line and catheter and also be there to balance on while you regain your strength, you will be able to do it. This can feel very silly at first and is much harder than it sounds. It can leave you feeling pretty drained and even dizzy. However, it's the first major important step towards your healing. As hard as it is, be strong for you and your baby. Getting up and moving around often, even in small little motions, is going to drastically speed up your recovery! The sooner you are able to get up and walk, the sooner your body can start to heal and also begin to process the abdominal gas that gathers internally after your surgery. This abdominal gas often has the potential to cause a lot of pain after your surgery, especially if it moves up into your shoulders. It's also important to keep your body moving so that your blood can continue circulating well. This goes a long way in decreasing the risk of a blood clot as your body begins to heal.

In addition to the nurses checking on your wellbeing, they'll also be coming in to check on the baby's vitals, too. Be prepared for a lot of interruptions in your room!

The Day After Your Cesarean

Your catheter will likely be removed the day after your cesarean, although depending on the time your surgery took place, it may come out sooner. It doesn't hurt to have it removed, although it does feel a little weird! It only takes a quick moment to get it out, so don't stress too much about this part. Having it out will make you feel like a new woman! Keep in mind though that you are now solely responsible for walking to and from the bathroom as needed! This is actually a good thing as it gives you a good excuse to continue moving around instead of just lying flat in bed the whole time.

Usually, they'll also remove your IV within twenty-four hours of your surgery. It will feel so amazing to have your hand and arm fully available to handle your baby without an extra line attached. Again, it doesn't hurt to have it removed; it's more like a quick little pinch. By this point, you'll also have received an oral pain medication that you can take every four to six hours on schedule. Definitely stay on top of this so that you can continue to move around. This is also a good time to start wearing your abdominal support band, too, which will help with moving around and caring for your baby.

The second day is when some women complain of having excruciating gas pains. These can be particularly bad in your shoulders. When your bowels become sluggish after surgery, gas can press on your diaphragm, triggering a nerve and extending the pain to the shoulders. Some women complain of this symptom lasting for several days. Applying peppermint essential oil is the only thing I have found that actually helped lessen this pain.

The nurses will likely check on you and the baby a little less as the day advances. They will still do occasional blood pressure and temperature tests, but it will not be as frequent as it was earlier. This is usually a great chance for you and baby to get some rest!

Two Days After Your Cesarean

You and your baby will likely be discharged from the hospital on day three. You may be in a hurry to get home, or you may be overwhelmed at the thought of managing both you and your baby at home all on your own. I have experienced both of those feelings as well as landing somewhere in between. It is overwhelming to think of going home with bandages on your incision, a new baby, and a body that hardly knows how to move properly. Trust me, it will be okay! This is the part where it is completely okay to reach out to friends and family for support. Do not be scared to open up to others with the reservations you are having. Have your husband or support partner help you wherever they can and try to be completely honest with them as to what they can do to make things easier for you.

Before you leave the hospital, you'll also be required to fill out a ton of discharge paperwork, as well as speak to a nurse about what you can expect when going home and what signs you should watch for that could potentially indicate an infection.

I strongly recommend wearing your abdominal support band on the way home as well as having an extra pillow to hold on your lap in the vehicle. This will make going over bumps and through turns a little bit easier. Even something as simple as car movements can make it feel like your tummy is all over the place during the first few days!

The Next Six Weeks

I considered breaking up the timeline into even smaller increments than six weeks; however, it just didn't seem to make sense. As I replayed all of my past cesareans and tried to organize a proper timeline of healing after I arrived home, I realized that every single one was completely different from the others, and yours will be too. My first cesarean was by far the worst. It felt as though it took months before I started feeling like myself again. With my last three cesareans, I felt like I was up and running after the first week despite a NICU stay, a snowstorm, and navigating life with a newborn during the covid pandemic. Your healing timeline will no doubt have your own bumps and quirks; however, I do promise that if you take the time to listen to your body and to truly take care of yourself, you will soon be up and on the move and settling into this new stage of motherhood just perfectly.

How you heal will depend on your body, your baby, the rest you are able to get, and many other circumstances surrounding your recovery period. The best advice I can give is to get as much rest as you possibly can! Walk around often, but do not overdo it if you start to feel pain, dizziness, or exhaustion. One thing that was fairly common in all my deliveries was that I always felt like I had a major setback somewhere between day ten and day fourteen. This occurs because that's often about the time you start to feel much better, so you naturally become very excited to start doing a lot of the things you haven't been able to do in a long time. Without even thinking about it, you stretch yourself far beyond your capabilities, which in turn can make you burn out pretty quickly. Even once you start to feel better, remember to take it slowly and ask for help whenever you can. It's better to heal slowly than to try to speed things up, which will only set you back in the future.

A Few Things to Keep in Mind During Your Six-Week Post-Recovery Period

- Do not lift anything heavier than your baby.
- Stay on top of your medication until you feel your body is ready to function without it.
- Get as much rest as you possibly can.
- Walk small distances often to keep your body moving, help your body relieve the abdominal gas, and keep your blood circulating well.
- Take advantage of your abdominal support band. Use it whenever you need to move around the house or even when you sleep. It will make turning around in bed so much easier and even allow you to slowly sleep back on your tummy if you prefer! Just remember to go without it at times, too, so your incision can breathe and get some fresh air.
- Apply colloidal silver gel to your incision daily. This can help in preventing an infection, and it can also assist with speeding up your recovery.
- When showering, try to avoid harsh soaps. Rather, stick to a mild soap and simply allow the warm water to run down your body and over your incision. You do not need to scrub your incision. Be sure to dry this area thoroughly after each shower.

- Avoid bathing until you are certain you can climb in and out of the tub with ease. For many moms, this is usually after 2 weeks. That first bath you have will feel amazing and is totally worth the wait!

- Keep your baby as close to you as possible during the first little while to make transitioning around the home easier.

- Eat a well-balanced diet to ensure both you and your baby are getting the nutrition you need.

- Drink a LOT of water! And then drink some more!

- No sex until you are cleared by your doctor. You don't want to cause any internal damage.

- Watch for signs of an infection such as redness or swelling at the incision site, pus or discharge by your incision, pain that is constantly getting worse, body chills, or foul smelling vaginal discharge. If you are unsure, you should always consult with your doctor immediately. Do not wait for your six-week postpartum checkup if you feel something is not right.

- Make sure you go in for your six-week postpartum checkup, even if you are feeling well!

And most importantly, enjoy this time with your baby! Say no to company if you need. Don't worry about the house chores. Use this time to bond with your baby and get to know the new little life you just brought home! You will have time for all of the other stuff later... and it really does go by fast!

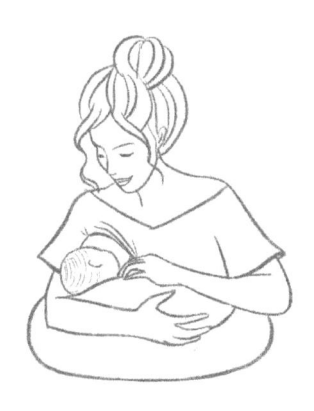

CHAPTER 10
Breastfeeding

How to overcome the difficulties of
breastfeeding while healing from a cesarean.

I REALLY DON'T BELIEVE there is a single time in your life when you will ever receive more "helpful" advice (I mean that very, VERY sarcastically!) then immediately after the birth of your first baby! Between sleep schedules, how to properly dress them, whether you should swaddle or not, and especially when it comes to breastfeeding, you'll have heard it all by the time your baby's first few months have come and gone! Sure, some of it will be welcomed and is actually helpful. However, more often than not—even if it is given by someone who means well—it can cause confusion, stress, uneasiness, and feelings of being overwhelmed. You are the mama, and just like every other mother before you, you will figure it out. After all, no one has ever raised your specific baby with your specific personality under your specific circumstances.

Breastfeeding your baby falls deep into this category, too. If you're looking for specific help when it comes to feeding your baby, the hospital always has lactation specialists on hand who will meet with you at the hospital. You can also plan to meet with them either by phone or in person once you return home from the hospital as well. Leave the breastfeeding advice up to the professionals or at least to trusted friends who have truly walked this journey before you.

Some of the first "recommendations" I heard both from family and some of the nursing staff after I delivered my first baby by cesarean were anything but helpful. They said things like breastfeeding would be much more difficult because of my surgery, and how my milk supply would take longer to come in because of the anesthesia I had. Some even said I should strongly consider supplementing with formula until my pain improved because it was more important for me to rest. The worst of all was when I was told I should completely give up the idea of breastfeeding and focus instead on healing my body so I didn't have to worry about the baby's weight gain or struggling through the night with difficult feedings! *Right!* Who wants to hear that right after having a baby?!

All of those statements couldn't have been further from the truth, and they were definitely not what I wanted to hear after just being released from surgery, especially since the cesarean came as a complete surprise. In fact, breastfeeding immediately after your cesarean is the absolute fastest way to heal from your surgery and also the best way to bond with your new baby. Of course, there may be scenarios when breastfeeding is not an immediate or future option for you or your baby. In these cases, I suggest working with your doctors and lactation specialists to figure out your next course of action. However, it truly *is* possible in most situations, and if you are able to, I definitely suggest pushing through all of the difficulties at the beginning. It will be totally worth it in the future.

Nurses, friends, and many other caring people in my life were not even intending to be disheartening or rude; they were just repeating common misconceptions they had heard in the past. There used to be a time when the pain medication they offered for surgery was not recommended during breastfeeding. However, since then this has completely changed, and unless your doctor has prescribed you something outside of the normal protocol, the pain medication they put you on after your surgery is completely fine for breastfeeding.

According to the CDC,[3] less than 50% of mothers exclusively breastfeed past three months. It also states that nearly 20% of all infants receive formula supplementation by their second day of life. As a new mother's milk can take anywhere from three to five days to fully come in, this indicates to me that mothers are often made to feel their supply is inadequate, even within the first few days of their babies' lives. However, the majority of babies are more than okay to start off their first days with only a small amount of colostrum. Of course, if there's a medical reason to supplement, I would never want to deny that opportunity to a baby in need. I just wonder if between a strong push from their medical team and well-meaning friends and family, new mothers are not receiving enough encouragement, assistance, and patience when it comes to nourishing their babies with their own breastmilk.

So, How Should I Get Started Breastfeeding My Baby After Surgery?

Breastfeeding your baby is optimal for healing as it allows your uterus to contract back to its original size much more quickly. In fact, you will actually feel it contracting every time your baby

---

3   https://www.cdc.gov/breastfeeding/data/facts.html

latches and starts to feed. Aren't our bodies amazing? Sometimes this can be slightly painful, while other times it actually feels quite healing. Be prepared to use lot of pads in your underwear, especially while feeding. As mentioned earlier, some women don't realize that you bleed vaginally even after a cesarean. Every time your uterus shrinks a little, it will also have extra blood that it needs to get rid of. Being prepared *down below* will keep both your clothes and your sheets in check a little longer.

If you feel comfortable immediately after your surgery, definitely ask to hold your baby as much as you can. After all of my surgeries except for one, I was able to hold my baby right away; although there were always periods when I had to pass him or her back to Dad for a break. Don't do anything that doesn't feel comfortable to you. If you are still feeling anxious or weak from the surgery, it's okay to wait until your body relaxes a little more. As soon as you are able, you'll want to get your baby skin to skin with you, and then onto your breast. This can be done as soon as you are comfortable, even while you are in the recovery room.

If for any reason your baby has complications and requires more care from the medical staff or needs to be transferred into the NICU, you'll want to use a pump as soon as you get the opportunity. You can ask for one the minute they move you into your room. I have included more details about the NICU and pumping in Chapter 11.

With the exception of my fifth and sixth baby, who were both admitted into the NICU for a short period of time, I did not need to pump or supplement a single one of them with formula, and my milk supply always started to come in around two to three days after surgery, with its full surge coming in around day four or five. As long as you continue to put the baby on your breast often, at two- to three-hour intervals during the day and then three- to five-hour intervals during the night, your supply should come in on a fairly similar timeline.

After your cesarean, you'll likely find that your baby is quite tired and more likely to fall asleep at the breast. This is totally okay! Rather than becoming frustrated that they tire easily and have such little energy to practice their latch, focus on enjoying this time of snuggling with your newborn, and take advantage of the extra rest time you can squeeze in. Even just having them skin to skin and close to your chest will do wonders for increasing your milk-producing hormones and working towards initiating your supply.

One thing you can do to make your baby more interested in the breast is to extract your colostrum with your fingers and rub it along their lips and on the roof of their mouth. This will help them become interested in feeding sooner. If they continue to drift off to Wonderland, you can also lightly tickle the sides of their mouth and cheeks with your fingers to entice them to wake up again. If they refuse to wake up, let them fall back asleep and try again in a few hours.

When Should I Worry About My Baby Gaining Weight After Birth?

It is normal for babies to lose up to 10% of their birth weight within the first few days after delivery, and then it usually takes between ten and fourteen days for them to reach their birth weight again. If your baby is still not gaining weight within the recommended timeframe, you should talk to your doctor. However, when a baby is newly born, they are learning right alongside you, and they are still used to spending the majority of their days and nights asleep. Rather than focus on how long your baby is staying awake on your breast, focus on how often you place him or her on the breast and spend a lot of time just holding him or her close by. Do not let the preconceived notion that they are not getting enough to eat cause you to become worried and stressed over your milk supply. Babies' tummies are so small. In that first day, all they require is the tiniest bit of colostrum to get their systems going. As your colostrum increases and slowly turns into more and more milk, their tummies start to grow just at the right time. It really is amazing how well we are designed!

How Often Should I Put My Baby on the Breast After They Are Born?

Try to have your baby on your breast at least every two to three hours during the day, and then every three to five hours during the night. Don't rush these first feeding sessions, and feel free to clear the room of any staff or visitors if you are the type who likes to learn in more of a quiet environment. Of course, some staff may be very helpful, but if you find that you are simply getting more stressed when they are in the room, kindly ask them to give you some quiet time and come back later. This is your baby, and you do not need to feel obligated to have them hovering over you and baby while you are still learning. *(I am speaking directly from experience here!)*

Most of my babies slept very well the first few nights after they were born, and you may find this is the scenario for you and your baby, too. This often happens with cesarean babies. If they are still sleeping after four or five hours in the night, you will, however, want to wake them up for a feeding session just to keep working on your supply. A good time to do this is when the nurse comes in to check you and your baby's vitals or obviously when your baby starts to wake up. However, if your baby is asleep in the night and it has only been a few hours and you are able to get some extra rest, do not worry about waking them up if it has been less than five hours since you last had them on your breast. You'll have plenty of time to put them on the breast during the day. Rest plays a vital role in bringing in your milk supply, and if you are lucky enough to catch a few extra hours during the night, take it!

Is There Anything I Can Do to Speed Up My Milk Fully Coming In?

The quick answer is: YES! Most, if not all, health food stores offer lactation teas and supplements that can greatly increase your milk supply. These range from vitamins, herbs, and powders that you can add to your yogurts, cereal, oatmeal, or soups. I highly recommend purchasing these in advance and adding them to your diet while at the hospital. Continue their use at home, too, at least until you feel you have a strong supply and a good handle on breastfeeding. The teas are actually very relaxing and a nice change from the sometimes weak or not-so-appealing alternatives they offer at the hospital.

Rest also plays a huge role in breastfeeding. While you're in the hospital healing, as well as your first days or weeks at home, take as much time as you can to rest. I know this is easier said than done between visits, baby needs, and other responsibilities. Don't feel bad for telling well-meaning visitors to wait a few extra days or asking friends and family for help if needed. Remember that the more prepared you are at home for bringing your baby home, the easier it will be to find those few quiet moments of rest. I promise, soon enough your supply will come in strong and heavy, and you will likely have more milk than you know what to do with!

How Can I Hold and Nurse My Baby if My Abdomen is Still So Uncomfortable from My Surgery?

I am not going to lie; breastfeeding after your surgery can be quite uncomfortable and requires even more creativity than if your baby was born vaginally. Even something as simple as reaching into their bassinet to lift the baby over the rail and into your bed can cause quite a bit of pain and even some dizziness in the beginning. The effort it takes to sit or stand up, reach in, and pick up your baby can be quite draining in the first few days. Even simple things like shuffling your butt towards the back of your bed to sit up straight can be exhausting. Although you can definitely take advantage of the adjustment buttons on the hospital bed, you might find that no matter what you try, it can be very hard getting into comfortable positions. This is the first reason why I highly recommend every cesarean mom has a good abdominal support band to put on as soon as possible after surgery, along with a comfortable breastfeeding pillow to rest and elevate your baby while feeding.

An abdominal support band quickly became an invaluable tool in my post-cesarean recovery period, and once I experienced the benefits after my second cesarean, I would never want to be without. Because I was not expecting to have a cesarean with my first baby, I did not have one available in the hospital or at home after my son's birth. Everything was almost unbearable, from standing up to turning around in bed to laughing or crying. For every cesarean afterwards, I made sure I had one packed in my hospital bag. As soon as I was able to get up and walk without assistance, I would gently place the abdominal support band around the bandages of my incision.

You'll want to make sure you take the band off often so your incision can get some air. Because the nurses will be checking on you quite regularly, this is generally a good time to remove it. Having abdominal support during breastfeeding allowed me to move around quicker, reach for my baby, and shift positions with very little discomfort. It also made it nice during the times when my husband wasn't able to be in the room, allowing me to take care of my new baby with much more ease. Having a support band will even make things like laughing and sneezing much more enjoyable.

Some abdominal supports are better than others, and some are specifically made for cesareans. Definitely take the time to read reviews and choose accordingly. I promise you that they are worth the investment. I spent quite a lot of money on my first one, which was specifically geared towards a cesarean recovery, and it has held up perfectly through all of my cesareans. It even came with a separate piece that attached to the front of the band just to tighten everything in a little more thoroughly over the incision. Just remember to size up when ordering, as you will still likely look and feel fairly pregnant at the beginning and also have extra swelling from the surgery! (Don't worry, it goes away faster than you think!)

I also suggest having a comfortable breastfeeding pillow with you at the hospital to help hold and elevate the baby. It will make things work much more smoothly for you, and it also acts as a restful place for the baby to lie while you get your shirt open or pulled down and everything else in place to feed the baby.

Whether you are still at the hospital or in the first early weeks at home, I suggest you also make sure you have a bedside table very close by where you can store snacks, burp clothes, diapers, wipes, lip gloss, and a gigantic water bottle. Every time I have been at the hospital, they've always had a little table with wheels that I could move right beside my bed. If you have this option, definitely take advantage of it. It's the perfect place to store everything you'll need without having to have a nurse or support partner (who will not always be available) pass you the things you require.

You have not experienced thirst like you will experience after your cesarean and during the early stages of breastfeeding. Even with the largest water bottle beside my bed, I could not keep it filled! My husband was constantly running around to fill it up with ice and water, both at the hospital and at home. Make sure you have plenty of water available and close by before you begin your breastfeeding sessions.

As mentioned earlier, one of the positive things about a cesarean is that you get to have a catheter in for the first twelve to twenty-four hours after surgery. I know this sounds crazy, and yes, at times they are pretty uncomfortable. The idea of a catheter used to freak me out, too. However, since you have to have it in anyways, you might as well enjoy the fact that, unlike the last month of pregnancy when you had to run to the bathroom after even the tiniest sip of water, you are now free to drink as much as you want without having to go to the bathroom at all. Drinking a ton of water is extremely beneficial to having a strong milk supply. So, drink away knowing that the catheter will take care of any extra water for now. Win-win in my book!

Before they remove your catheter, you'll likely have already walked to and from the bathroom several times with your catheter bag and IV line in tow. For the first few times you are required to get up and walk, you'll likely be hanging onto your support partner, nurse, or the side of the bed while you attempt to get up. Although this will feel very exhausting at first, you'll feel amazing just walking around a little. And once you are able to have your catheter removed, you can put on your own clothes and breastfeed and care for your baby in something that feels a little more human. You will be on your way to feeling much more like yourself.

As soon as they remove your catheter, you'll be able to change out of your hospital gown and into something more comfortable. This is a draining and difficult task, so be prepared. Leggings or shorts with a high waist that offers compression was always the most comfortable clothing for me. Pairing those with a tighter tank top that can open easily for breastfeeding was also my preferred choice. Others might prefer having looser clothes that don't rub against your incision, and often this is a recommendation you may receive from your doctor or see listed on many cesarean pamphlets. I always found that I was constantly shifting positions while breastfeeding or moving around to change the baby's diaper, so the less likely I was to be tangled among the bed sheets, the better. I generally found that loose clothes got more twisted up and made it quite difficult for me to get comfortable. As long as your incision is well bandaged up, having clothing up against your waist might actually feel good to you like it did for me. Just remember to pull the waistband of your leggings down several times a day to let your incision air out. The more often you give your wound some fresh air, the faster it will start to heal!

Once your milk supply comes in full force (and I mean with a vengeance), nursing pads will also become a life-saver and will soon become your best friend! For the first little while after surgery, you will be most comfortable sleeping on your back. However, you will likely move onto your side or tummy as soon as you feel up to it. It feels *so* good to finally be able to sleep on your tummy again after being pregnant for nine months, but it is uncomfortable to wake up in the night with milk puddles in the sheets and blankets. While your milk supply is establishing itself, you'll notice when it comes in that it will come in heavy and all at once without any warning at all. If you are in a deep sleep, you will not even notice it leaking out. The last thing you want to do while healing from surgery is to have to change your sheets in the middle of the night. I can testify that this is NOT AT ALL FUN, even with the help of your husband! Having a good breastfeeding bra and good quality nursing pads is vitally important and should not be overlooked.

Burping the Baby

Pregnancy was not a sprint and neither is breastfeeding. The best things in life are often the most amount of work. When it comes to breastfeeding your new baby, one of the most important things you can do to make your baby comfortable is to take your feeding sessions slowly, while patiently burping your baby immediately after their feed or even several times during their feed. Getting in and out of bed with your baby is tricky enough after your cesarean. You might as well take the extra time to make sure that all of their needs are met before you attempt to lay them back down. Although burping babies between and after feeds is common breastfeeding practice, I want to emphasize the importance of getting out that extra air often, even if it takes a while.

I always found that for me the most comfortable position to burp a baby without hurting my incision was to have them sit on a pillow that is protecting your abdomen while they have their chin leaning into your hand. Use your other hand to lightly pat and massage their backs. If they are having trouble burping, gently lean them forwards and backwards and then pat and massage them again until they burp. Training your new little baby to burp often during breastfeeding will help prevent air blockages, which in turn can affect the rest of their feeds and the sleep that follows. I can remember taking up to twenty minutes or more sometimes just to get out a little, tiny burp. I was tired and exhausted and wanted nothing more than for my baby's tummy to fill up so that we could both fall back asleep. However, if you miss or rush this very important step, you'll often be woken up only moments later with an uncomfortable baby who is full of gas, or a baby who was not fed properly because they were too filled up with air to eat their entire feed.

You want to ensure that they are filling up on milk rather than air, and it will also make them more comfortable when you put them back down to sleep. It is better to take a longer, more relaxed approach to feeding and have your baby sleep much better afterwards than it is to rush through the feed and have them fuss as soon as you put them down. This process will speed up over time and soon your baby will become a pro-burper and pro-feeder. Just remember that for now, they are still training and learning what life is like on the outside, just like you are learning what life is like as a new mother. Don't rush them. Have patience and let time be your guide.

The Painful or Not-So-Comfortable Parts of Breastfeeding

Many women also struggle with sore and cracked nipples during the beginning of their breastfeeding journey. I know a lot of women, including myself, who found relief in some of the natural nipple creams that are available to purchase. For me, I went back and forth using those creams or applying colloidal silver gel to simply extracting colostrum at the beginning and rubbing it around the breast. These all worked great at helping the nipples feel a little bit better in the early stages. Definitely pack these along in your hospital bag to make the transition easier.

Around day three, four, or maybe even five, your milk will likely be coming in strong and steady. This is often the most painful part of breastfeeding, and a time when a lot of mothers want to give up. On one hand, you are excited that you finally have a strong supply of milk for your baby, while on the other hand, it's coming out so fast and your breasts are so engorged that it makes it fairly difficult for the baby to get a good latch, let alone eat without nearly feeling like they are choking on the milk! If your breasts are too full, you can often hand express some of the extra milk in the shower or in the sink. Just make sure you don't express too much as our bodies work on a supply-and-demand basis, and the more milk that is taken out, the more our bodies will want to produce to keep up with the demand.

As hard as it is, I promise that over the next few days and weeks, you and your baby will find a flow and rhythm that works well for the both of you. While your milk supply is flowing with such force, it is super important to take breaks and allow your baby to catch their breath in between. Burp your baby, rub their back, and make sure you are telling them what a wonderful job they are doing. It will get easier for both of you. If you find that you are still having problems with breastfeeding, this might be an excellent time to book a consultation with a lactation specialist. They are seriously beyond amazing in supporting and offering you all kinds of encouragement and tips to help you along the way.

If breastfeeding is something that is extremely important to you, there are actually very few reasons as to why you cannot make this your reality, even with a cesarean. Sure, it might require more strength and can be more painful at the beginning, but I want to encourage you and assure you that the way you feel at the beginning is shorter lived than you might realize. It is well worth every bit of effort.

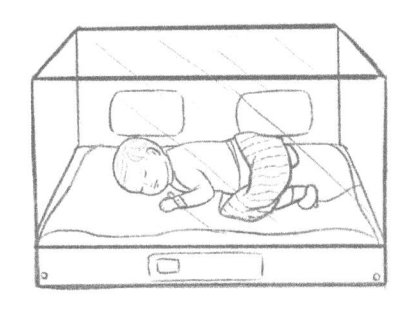

CHAPTER 11
NICU Baby

What to expect if your new baby requires
time in the NICU after your cesarean

WHEN I WAS thirty-six weeks pregnant with my fifth child, I started to have more Braxton Hicks contractions than I remembered having with my other babies. I knew they were really common in the last trimester, particularly as you get closer to the end of your pregnancy and your body begins its preparation for labor. However, something was different this time. They seemed to be coming more and more often, especially during the night. Many nights I would get up and start timing them for several hours until they calmed down, and I would fall back asleep. As the days progressed, they began to happen for hours at a time during the day, too. I decided to make a special appointment to see my OB/GYN just to have her reassure me that everything was all right. I was already scheduled for a cesarean just past thirty-eight weeks, but the doctors were not keen on me having too many contractions, simply because of the number of cesareans I had already had. Of course, when I went into my appointment, absolutely all of the contractions completely stopped. They monitored me for over an hour and were not able to see anything, so they sent me home and told me to go straight to the hospital for monitoring if it happened again.

The very next day, the contractions started up again in the morning. As the day went on, they definitely got stronger and more intense. By late afternoon, I decided that I wanted to go to the hospital for reassurance. My husband and I did not have a sitter for the other four kids, so we took the whole family for a drive. He dropped me off at the front doors and decided to take the kids for some snacks while I was monitored. After about an hour of having the monitor on my belly, it was determined that I was, in fact, in labor, and they wanted to deliver the baby by cesarean within the next few hours. My husband was pretty surprised when I called him and told him to take the kids home to their grandparents, grab the hospital bags, and come back as quickly as he could. (This is another reason why it is always good to be prepared in advance!) I actually had most of the kids' things already to go, which made it much easier for him to organize in a hurry. Within two hours, my husband had fed the kids supper, dropped them off with their grandparents, packed up the bags, and returned to the hospital. It was go time!

Although I was super excited to meet this little guy, it was an extra week earlier than we had planned to have the cesarean. The doctors informed that although some babies are fine, others may require a short time in the NICU. The NICU (Neonatal Intensive Care Unit) is a specialized care unit that is specifically for ill or premature newborns. If your baby was born too early, has an underlying health condition, or had any complications during the delivery, they will likely require some extra attention in the NICU. Although it sounds completely intimidating at first, having your baby in the NICU is the safest place for them to be in order to get the twenty-four-hour care that is required while healing. My hopes were high that all would be fine, and we moved into the surgery room for delivery.

As soon as he was born, they checked his vitals and then placed him in my arms. To me, he seemed perfect. I don't think I noticed that his color was a bit off or that he was having a bit of trouble taking deep breaths. After a few moments, one of the NICU doctors came over to check his vitals again and within a few short moments, he was taken away to the NICU with very little explanation to me or my husband as to what was going on. All they kept on saying was that they would call us with an update once they had more information. It was AWFUL! I was not the least bit prepared to have my son taken away, and I honestly didn't think it would happen to us. My heart was broken, and I felt like part of me had been ripped away.

Although most soon-to-be moms never put much thought into the possibility, roughly between 10% and 15% of all births require at least a short stay in the NICU after delivery. Unfortunately for cesarean deliveries, that number is slightly higher. Having a baby in the NICU after a vaginal birth is difficult enough on its own. However, having a baby taken to the NICU directly after the mama has undergone a cesarean delivery can cause an entirely new set of challenges. After all, you'll still be attached to both your catheter and IV, which can make moving around much more difficult. Taking your catheter bag and IV bag down to an entirely new floor while you have just come out of surgery will be difficult, if not nearly impossible. You may be required to wait until the catheter and IV are removed before you are able to visit your baby again.

I know this sounds hard. And it is. It was actually the worst part for me and probably will be for you, too. After all, you have just carried this precious baby for your entire pregnancy only to have them whisked away only moments after you've just met. This is just another instance where your husband or support partner becomes invaluable. Since they are actually able to move around the hospital and carry on calmer conversations with the medical team, they will be your rock as you head into this new journey. As soon as your baby is settled in their NICU bed, the staff will allow your support partner to visit and likely get a much clearer picture of what is going on. This is an excellent time for them to take pictures, videos, and make phone calls back up to Mama to make sure you feel included in the entire process. Most NICUs are also extremely helpful in taking phone calls from Mom and answering any questions that you may have. Don't feel like you are an inconvenience. They are actually set up to make the process as easy as possible, and they have staff and nurses set aside to answer any questions that you may have. If your baby's nurse is busy at the time, they will always call you back when they have an update.

I wish I could sugar-coat what it really feels like to not be with your baby immediately after delivery, but I can't. It's such an emotional experience. Holding your baby after the cesarean makes everything about what you have just been through seem much easier to deal with. There is an indescribable strength that a mom gets when they feed their baby for the first time, or when they look into their newborn's eyes when they open in the wee hours of the night. And now it will feel like you are all alone. And on top of dealing with your emotions, you will be completely worried for your precious baby who is in a completely new bed, new floor, and away from his mom. It is okay to cry... *like a lot*. It is okay to be upset and grieve what you expected it would be like to meet your new baby. It will feel like so much has been taken away from you, and it will seem impossible to know what to do next. But I promise, it gets easier.

In this moment, it might even feel easy to turn your emotions, possibly even anger, towards the health-care team working with your baby. Trust me. I have totally been there. It feels in that moment that you should be the sole provider for your infant, not some seemingly cold doctors and nurses. As difficult as this will be, you will be in better shoes if you can at least start off on a good foot with the medical team responsible for the care of your baby. Remember they are there to help you and your baby, and their main goals are actually the exact same as yours—to get baby healthy and home as soon as possible.

So, what should you do now that you are back in your recovery room without your baby? Start by taking care of yourself first. A healthy mom makes for a healthy baby. Don't rush the most important and healing steps of recovering from your cesarean. Eat well, drink plenty of water, and let the nursing staff take care of your needs. Now is the time to focus on getting as strong as you can so that you can be present and alert for the care of your new baby. Sometimes this will mean pushing yourself to walk more or to make healthier food choices so that you recover more quickly, while other times this will mean taking the time to rest when you know are overdoing it, even though you want nothing more than to spend every waking minute with your baby.

The most healing, difficult, and strengthening thing that I did to help me get through the first few days of healing in the hospital was to start pumping immediately after they took me back to my room. Most hospitals will provide you with an amazing hospital-grade pump and all of the supplies required, including anything that is needed to wash and rinse the reusable parts. They will likely have them available both in your room as well as in the NICU so that wherever you are at the moment, you can always pump as often as you would like. You will also have a designated area in the fridge or freezer of the NICU where they will allow you to store your pumped and labelled milk as soon as you or your support partner are able to start bringing it down. As soon as you get even the tiniest drop of colostrum, you'll want to bottle it up and send it over to your baby. If your baby is already able to have breastmilk, the NICU staff will be more than happy to give it to your baby as soon as they are able. If your baby is still too small to eat from a bottle but ready to tolerate some breastmilk or colostrum in their tummies, they will likely need to offer this through a form of tube feeding.

Some babies are too little to have any breastmilk or formula in the early stages. If this is the case with your baby, the nursing staff will be more than happy to help you store it for future use. Breastmilk is so important for newborn babies, but it plays an even more crucial role when your baby is in the NICU because it is so full of vital nutrients, hormones, and other growth factors. It will go a long way in helping prevent infections, as well as to protect them from other viruses or respiratory issues that they may be more susceptible to. It is also much easier to digest than formula, which is especially important when their digestive systems are still so small and only learning to function.

Building up your milk supply and bringing in your milk during those first few days is really quite similar to breastfeeding your new baby. Having amazing supplements, a good diet, and pumping often are all vital in setting the stage for successful breastfeeding. The only difference is that you will not have a hungry baby telling you when it is time to feed. This is where it is crucial to set yourself up on a schedule and try to stick to it as closely as you can. Ideally, pumping every three hours is optimal, or about eight times in a twenty-four-hour period. I preferred pumping a little more often during the day and trying to get in at least one four- to five-hour stretch in the night. This never seemed to affect my milk. In fact, all of my babies (including the two who had a short stay in the NICU) successfully breastfed until at least their first birthday.

Once your catheter and IV are removed, you'll likely be jumping at the chance to go down and meet your baby again. Depending on the layout of your hospital, you'll very likely want to have someone take you down in a wheelchair for those first few visits. Even if it feels like you are walking quite steadily already, those hospital floors are cold and hard, and it may be a fairly big deal to get from your room all the way down to the NICU. You may need to wait to be let into the room or to speak with doctors first. Having a wheelchair is a great way to save up your energy for spending time with your precious baby. It can also be a very emotional experience seeing your baby hooked up to all of those extra cords and monitors at first. If you've been standing too long, you may become dizzy or nauseous. Having a wheelchair will be safest, and before long, your energy will be back, and you will be much more ready to be hands-on with your little one. But for now, while you are in the earliest stages of healing, take the time to rest whenever you can.

Remember to wear your abdominal band when you are moving around the hospital. It'll serve as the most helpful tool when visiting your newborn. If they allow you to hold your baby when you arrive, it's also very helpful to ask for a pillow to rest the baby on to separate the baby from your incision even more. Your baby will likely be attached to several monitors, which makes moving him or her around even more difficult. The pillow will just make it more comfortable for everyone.

> **Quick Tip:** Remember to go pee BEFORE you head over to visit baby. Getting settled in the NICU after a cesarean is a bit of a challenge. Nothing is worse than the nursing staff helping you settle your baby in your arms after what seems like an eternity of getting all the chords untangled only to find your bladder is completely full moments after you are handed your baby.

If you don't already have a good breast pump at home, using the time you're in the hospital to find one is a good idea. The NICU will provide one along with a quiet space for pumping while you are in the hospital, but you'll want something for when you go home, too. Although I had some basic pumps at home that worked in a pinch, I actually chose to rent the hospital-grade pumps you can get from the pharmacy for the first while until my baby was able to come home. Because I knew I would be solely relying on the pump to provide nutrition for my baby, I wanted something that was reliable, extremely efficient, quiet, and easy to use. They can be expensive, but in the end, for me it was still cheaper than purchasing a higher quality one when I knew I would only need it for a few weeks. If you do find that your baby requires a longer stay in the NICU, it may be more to your benefit to purchase a high-quality pump as opposed to renting one.

Be prepared for the day that they discharge you from the hospital... *without your baby*. Although some hospitals allow you to stay overnight with your baby in the NICU, many are simply not set up for Mom to stay the entire time. Yes, they let you visit anytime you like, but you'll want to get rest during the night so you can have the energy needed to take care of your baby during the day. The moment you leave the hospital without your baby can be very emotional. This is 100% not how you expected this to go. I bawled the whole way home. It's normal to feel like your soul has just been ripped out from under you. Go home, get some rest, take care of yourself, and breathe.

Once you're feeling a little less overwhelmed, you will have a much clearer headspace to start thinking about how to make the drive and visits to the hospital and back home a little bit easier. Have your support partner pack both of you some quality food to consume during the days, a bag with all of your pumping supplies so that you can transfer them easily back and forth, a comfortable pillow that you can relax with while hanging out in your baby's room, some cozy sweaters and walking shoes, and anything else you can think of to make your stay more enjoyable.

Most NICUs will also have a fridge where they allow parents to keep labelled food so you don't have to eat at the cafeteria all the time. Take a notebook, too, so you can record important information about your baby or write down questions you may have for your baby's medical team. It is very common to feel very clouded and overwhelmed after the birth of your baby, especially if they are now spending their first days, weeks, or even months in the NICU. It can be very difficult to remember everything that you are supposed to, so having a little travel notebook can do wonders for keeping you organized as you navigate this temporary stage of your life.

As difficult as it will be healing from your cesarean while visiting the NICU, I promise it will eventually pass. Your baby will become strong and healthy and will soon be in your arms in the comfort of your own home. My son came home after only one week of being in the NICU, and my daughter after two weeks. Even though that was such a short stretch of time compared to so many other babies, I can remember how cozy and beautiful it was to walk them through our front door and bring them home to meet their family. I literally spent the next few days doing almost nothing and just soaking it all in.

Having my babies in the NICU was one of the most difficult and yet most strengthening moments I have ever gone through as a mom, and yet I am happy it has become a small part of my story. I was able to meet so many amazing families and staff in the NICU, who I would never have met without those experiences. I am now able to comfort others who are in similar situations, and I have a new appreciation for everything that the medical team was able to do. You are every bit as strong and capable as any mother who has gone before you. You can do this, and you will. Because you are their mom!

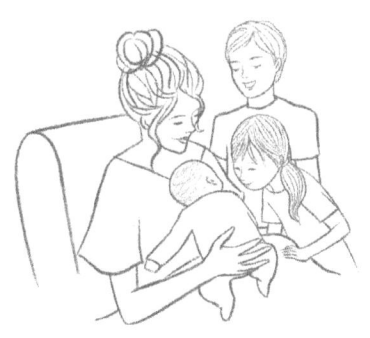

CHAPTER 12
First Week at Home

Realistic expectations for bringing your
baby home during the first week.

MAYBE YOU HAVE DONE everything right and feel that you are completely ready to take on the world once you arrive home with your new baby. Or maybe this cesarean came as a complete surprise, and you feel as though you have absolutely no idea what to expect when you are released from the hospital. Or even more likely, you are somewhere in between. That's okay! No matter how much you prepare in advance, there will always be unique challenges and circumstances surrounding your birth story.

As I mentioned earlier, about ten days after my first cesarean, my incision ended up opening up and becoming infected, which in turn required an emergency trip back to the hospital and hours and hours of being admitted with intravenous antibiotics. It was not a fun experience and actually very frightening in the moment. With my second cesarean, I was told I was having a little girl based on the twenty-two-week ultrasound we had earlier in the pregnancy. To my complete surprise, the doctor announced what a beautiful baby boy we had when they first introduced me to him after my cesarean. (This definitely made for some interesting hospital outfits and first baby pictures!) For my third and fourth cesareans, we were in the transition of moving within weeks after both surgeries. I have also had two babies end up in the NICU, one of whom was born during one of the worst snowstorms we had experienced in over a decade *and* during the start of the covid ordeal! The point is, no matter how well you lay out your plans, life will always change. The more you are able to embrace this season of new beginnings, the easier it will be for your body to heal.

Regardless of whether your baby was born vaginally or by cesarean, bringing a new baby home from the hospital is likely going to be one of the best moments you will experience in your life. The smell of your home, the music you have on your current go-to playlists, and the ambiance of your environment will all be ingrained in your memory, stamping that moment in time into the depths of your heart and soul. *To this day I can still hum along perfectly to the yogurt commercial theme song that was playing on the television commercials way too often as I learned to breastfeed my new baby in those first few weeks after bringing him home.*

It will also be a very emotional time, full of ups and downs, tears of joy, and tears of pain, mixed with intense bursts of energy followed by deep exhaustion that only a new mama will ever understand. Coming home from the hospital, regardless of how your baby was born, will definitely have its up and downs. However, if you are coming home from the hospital after a cesarean, it will have its completely own set of challenges. Everything from using the stairs to making meals, to going to the bathroom and showering requires much more effort during the first few days and weeks after your surgery. Even getting in and out of bed can feel like a workout, and with a baby that is still learning how to sleep, eat, and be awake at the proper times, this can all feel completely overwhelming.

If you already read through Chapter 4, you will likely have your home fairly prepared in advance, which will go a long way in making things a bit easier for you. But what is it really like to bring your new baby home with your abdomen all bandaged up and your ability to do normal household tasks completely challenged?

Well, that all depends on how your body is healing, what type of baby you have (no, you can't completely guarantee you'll have one who is quiet and restful all of the time), and other circumstances surrounding your due date. Unfortunately, babies do not come with one-size-fits-all instructions. Some of them will be amazing sleepers and perfect eaters right from day one. Others will buck the system a little more. Some will love sleeping independently in their own beds, while others will beg to be held more often than not. Some will have super-sensitive tummies and require more time learning to pass gas, while others will have this skill almost mastered from day one. There is no way I can guarantee for you exactly what your particular life will look like when you first walk in that door. Maybe your husband has taken time off from work and is able to assist you at every waking moment to take care of all of your needs. Or maybe he will be home for only a few days before heading out of town for work again. I have experienced both, and I can assure you that although one scenario is much easier than the next, I have survived both.

If you already have other children in the home, it becomes an entirely new process that can seem even more overwhelming, especially if you are not prepared ahead of time. However, after having seven cesareans, I can assure you that it is possible to enjoy your new little baby at home while still taking time to enjoy all of the other little people, too. It took me a few tries to figure it out, and each birth presented itself with its own unique challenges, but I do believe that as moms we have the inner strength and the wisdom to make it through these difficult moments. In fact, I would go as far as to say that it is in these difficult moments of vulnerability that we are able to grow in character and in patience. I had to realize that it is okay to sometimes be unable to do it all alone! It is okay to rest, completely okay to use disposable dishes for a while, okay to have screen-time run a little longer than normal for the kids, and definitely okay for you to feel like it is all falling apart in the meantime! I promise, it does get better—much better—and probably sooner than you expect.

There is no specific answer as to how you are going to feel the first week at home after your cesarean. Some moms report being up on their feet often and able to go for short walks with very little pain during the first week. Others report feeling completely exhausted with unbearable pain and finding it very difficult to care for their infant on top of everything crazy that is happening with their bodies. Both are normal. However, if you take the proper steps in caring for yourself, you can make huge strides to having the best healing timeline possible.

One of the most important things you can do when coming home from the hospital is to stay on top of your pain medication. I tend to be the type of person who will never take pain medication unnecessarily. In fact, I am probably one of the last people you would ask for a Tylenol or Advil because I generally like to let my body heal on its own or use other methods such as diet and supplements to help me get to the root of the problem. However, when it comes to taking pain medication post-surgery, I highly encourage you to stay on top of your prescriptions like clockwork. The most commonly prescribed medications are just regular Tylenol for the pain and Naproxen for the inflammation. The more you are able to stay on top of your pain management, the quicker you will be able to stop taking the medicine. If you skip taking them even for an hour or so, your pain can become fairly unmanageable, and it will be more difficult to get on back on track.

If your pain becomes too unbearable, it will likely make it much more difficult to walk around and take care of your baby. Movement helps your body heal much faster, and if you have so much pain that you restrict yourself to sitting or lying down for long periods of time, you actually will set your healing back quite a bit. With my first few cesareans, I needed to be on the painkillers for about ten days, while with others I was able to stop after about five to seven days. Once you are waking up at night with less and less pain, you will know that you can start to stretch out the amount of time in between each dose. Just be careful not to lay off too soon or wait too long in between your pain medication, or you can actually slow down your healing process.

One thing I always found super helpful was to have an ongoing list of medications and the times that they were last taken, either on my phone or in a journal. That way I could be sure I was staying on top of my pain management, even in the wee hours of the night. Although side effects are usually minimal and not too common with most pain medications, you will want to discuss with your doctor if you experience any uncomfortable symptoms, or if you find you are still having pain. Taking more than the recommended dosage or switching medications may not be safe for you or the baby unless it has been prescribed by your doctor.

Your incision is also something you'll want to keep clean and dry as best as you can. You will probably have staples or sterile strips directly on top of your incision that will help hold everything together. If you have staples, you may have a home nurse come over to remove them after the first few days, or you may be required to make a trip back to the hospital to have them removed. If you have the sterile strips on top instead (which is actually the most common method), they will slowly fall off over time. If you have the opportunity to ask, I highly recommend the sterile strips. They are much more comfortable. Regardless of how they bandage you up, keep a close eye on this area. You'll want to look for any signs of bleeding, pus, or red areas that feel hot to the touch. If you notice any of these signs, get in touch with your doctor to see what course of action they recommend. The longer you let these things go unaddressed, the more likely they are to lead to a more serious infection.

The first time I looked at my hanging and stitched-up stomach post-cesarean, I was completely freaked out. I honestly could not recognize anything. What on earth had just happened to it! It can look a little crazy at first with everything being loose, swollen, bruised, and cut up all at once, but I promise it does get better. Because I tend to lean on the side of squeamish when it comes to that kind of stuff, I always had my husband look at my incision for the first week to make sure it was healing up properly. After the first week or so, once my uterus had shrunk and the swelling started to go down, I was finally able to look at it myself without freaking out. Not everyone will be the same as me, and you may find it much more comfortable to just look at it yourself. Depending on your body, you may also have to lift up some of your swollen abdomen to be able to see the incision properly. Having a mirror also helps if you need to get a closer look. It is easy for water, pus, or blood to get trapped in that area if you do not keep a close eye on it. Simply lifting up your swollen abdomen in the shower, letting warm water run over it, and then patting it dry when you come out will do wonders.

As I mentioned earlier, an absolute must-have for healing from your cesarean is colloidal silver gel. If you remember anything from reading this book, it is the value of colloidal silver! I started using this after my second cesarean, and it is something that I'll never go without. Colloidal silver can be taken as a liquid or applied as a gel; it is a natural antibiotic that can do wonders in preventing an infection. It is also very soothing when applied to your incision. The doctors were always amazed at how fast my incisions healed, and I believe it's due to the consistent use of colloidal silver gel. I always started applying this gel on day two or three after my cesarean, directly on top of my incision. You can purchase colloidal silver at most natural health stores, or it can be ordered online either in liquid or gel form; no prescription required. Definitely add this to your healing regimen!

As mentioned earlier, wearing your abdomen support band as often as you can will also help speed up your recovery. This will make taking care of your baby so much easier. Most women who choose to use an abdominal support band continue to wear them for several weeks after coming home from the hospital. It makes everything easier.

I am sure by now you have probably heard the old saying: "Sleep when your baby sleeps." Although it does sound appealing, it is actually much easier said than done. If you are anything like me, you are going to find it difficult to rest if the dishes are staring at you, laundry piles are waiting for you, and kids are begging for your attention. This is where balance becomes so important. The more you can have your house prepared before you bring your baby home, the easier it will be to rest properly afterwards. However, there will definitely be times where you need to use the baby's nap time to catch up on some other tasks. Try to balance it out throughout the day. Maybe folding a load of baby blankets is tolerable in the morning, but then try to take some time in the afternoon to rest too.

If you have friends and family who are chafing at the bit to come over for a visit, be firm if you need to. You may be in a place where you can't wait to show off your new baby, or you might be so exhausted that you can't imagine visiting with anyone. I want to give you complete permission to be the boss of your home during this time. After all, it is *your* baby, *your* body, and *your* family. Don't hesitate to push friends and family off a little longer or at least minimize the amount of company if you feel you need the extra time to rest. Maybe you can handle a quick pop-over in the morning but would rather no afternoon or evening visits. That is okay!

Another thing you may want to consider is the time of year you are bringing your babies home. Five out of seven of my babies were born in winter when the flu and colds were in peak season. As idealistic as it may seem to send your kids away to play centers or public events, I always took the week leading up to delivery and the first two weeks after the cesarean to hunker down and stick close to home. Although you can't completely avoid being around germs, this is one of those times when you want to try and stay as healthy as possible. Dealing with sick kids, or a sick mama while healing from surgery is not fun!

If you can find friends and family to watch your kids for a few hours or maybe even days, it can be super helpful! However, make sure they are willing to keep your kids on a similar nap/sleep schedule as their normal routine so they are not falling apart at the seams when they return to you! Nothing is more difficult than sending your kids away for a break only to have them returned the next day more miserable and inconsolable than ever. This is especially important if your kids are under six years old. Having a new baby poses enough challenges and adjustments as it is; you do not want to add extra stress by having the siblings short on sleep, too.

Although you won't be able to get on the floor and play with your kids in the first few days and weeks like you could before, one thing I always did a lot after my cesareans was to read out loud to my kids. I have always cherished reading with my kids, but something about doing it with a new baby close by in a bassinet brings a sense of togetherness with the whole family. Choose books that everyone will enjoy. Another thing I often recommend is purchasing some new crayons, markers, or even pastels or paints to get out once the baby comes home. You might be surprised how long your kids will sit and create art, especially if you have a few new, exciting items to work with. And sitting down to color with them for a few moments is another way you can continue to fill up their love tank, which in return will make the transition of bringing a new baby home just a little bit easier. Chances are your kids will look back at this time and remember those precious moments over all of the other chaos.

Going for short walks if the weather allows is also an excellent way to pick up your spirits after bringing your baby home. Even a short time spent in a park or backyard can lift the entire family's mood. If you are still feeling like that is too much, definitely be sure not to overdo it. The last thing you want to do is to force your body to do something it is not ready for. You will know what your body is capable of each and every day.

The most important thing you can do is to relax! Order in pizza if you have to, let the dust bunnies hang out for a while, tell your friends to wait a little longer to visit if you need more time. It is all just fine! Do not let the greasy fingerprints on the walls or the smudges on your glass windows and mirrors stop you from enjoying your new baby and your precious family. Kids don't notice the mess in your home, but they will notice the mess in your heart if you allow yourself to become stressed out with what you cannot change. Let go of your need to have everything perfectly in place and embrace the sweet lives that you have been blessed to take care of.

> *"Love begins at home, and it is not how much we do… but how much love we put in that action."*
> —Mother Theresa

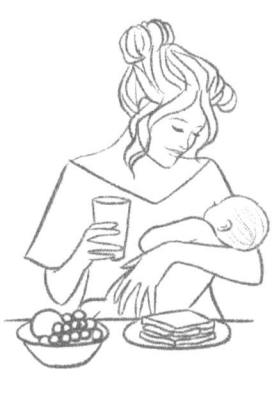

CHAPTER 13
Supplements, Diet, and Exercise for Healing

How to make the most of your pregnancy, cesarean, and postpartum healing through proper nutrition.

WHAT YOU EAT both during and after pregnancy matters. It matters for the health of your baby and for how quickly your body is able to heal after your cesarean. It also matters for how well you are able to establish and maintain a healthy breastfeeding supply. If you want to feel your best as a new mom and have the energy that is required for taking care of a new infant, you will not want to overlook proper nutrition. That is why I cannot stress enough that you need to be mindful of what you are putting into your body at all times, both during pregnancy and after you bring your baby home. Let's start off by talking about our hormones and how they affect pregnancy, labor, healing, and breastfeeding.

During pregnancy, our estrogen and progesterone levels shift quite substantially to allow our bodies to grow a baby. They slowly increase all the way until birth, when they hit their peak level to help our bodies prepare for labor. Since both our progesterone and estrogen are increased by the placenta, these hormones will drop dramatically once your baby is delivered. While this change is happening, our prolactin hormone goes into overdrive to signal our bodies that we need to start producing milk. Our oxytocin hormone, which is also called our "happy" hormone, is also going crazy as we fall madly in love with our new baby. All of these ups and downs can leave us feeling a bit unhinged for a while. Luckily, our bodies are incredible and amazing. When they are properly taken care of with good nutrition, things will generally begin to align themselves over time.

If you find you're struggling with your emotions and simply not feeling back to yourself, or if you start to feel depressed or anxious, you may want to speak with your health-care provider or talk to a friend or family member for support. Although many new moms will often experience some level of sadness after their baby is born, for others it can turn into something a little deeper. It is especially important to understand the differences between the *baby blues* versus *postpartum depression* as the treatment and timelines will differ.

When a mother experiences the baby blues after her baby is born, it is generally for a much shorter time period than with postpartum depression. It usually starts within a few days after giving birth and will subside within several weeks. Symptoms can include irritability, fatigue, sadness, anxiety, and feeling overwhelmed.

When a mother experiences postpartum depression, it is more likely to be noticed around four weeks or later and can last anywhere from a few months up to a year or more. Symptoms of postpartum depression can include extreme anxiety or stress, aggression, sadness that will not go away, anger, and potentially even feelings of detachment from the baby.

If you find yourself in either of these situations, definitely talk to a health-care provider. Know that it is not at all your fault—*in time, this too will pass*. Experiencing any form of depression does not mean that you are not a good mother. Many of the best moms that I have met have struggled with various levels of depression after their babies were born, and ALL of them have become some of the strongest, most compassionate, and most amazing human beings that I have ever met, who have unmeasurable love for their babies! Although you may feel like you are in a time or space that is completely disconnected from your family, your friends, your body, and your baby, you will eventually see the light and continue to thrive again. Sometimes we just need a little extra help or someone to talk to. Don't ever hesitate to ask for help if you feel something is not right.

More than likely, you'll feel an elevated sense of joy immediately after your baby is born. No matter how tired and exhausted you are from your surgery, you will probably feel relieved, energetic, and full of amazement with meeting your new little baby. And if you don't, that is perfectly okay, too. The amount of hormone fluctuations our bodies go through just to grow a tiny human is incredible. And the moment that baby is born, your hormones go through yet another incredible change while they adjust once again to love, support, and feed your baby. Adding a surgery on top of everything is just the icing on the cake! With all of my babies, I remember feeling so energized and excited, while at the same time completely deflated because of my surgery. It was difficult to move around and care for my baby the way I wanted to. This is a good time to let your partner pamper and support you. Also remember that your medical team is there to help you, too. Don't feel bad asking for help. Give your body some extra love, and don't be too hard on yourself. Every woman is affected differently. Be patient with this new phase and give yourself time to heal both emotionally and physically.

Proper nutrition during pregnancy and after pregnancy is SO important. Our bodies were not designed to be running on a sugar-laden and processed diet. As hard as it can be to maintain a healthy diet during and after pregnancy, we need to be sure to take care of ourselves to ensure our hormones have what they need to rebalance themselves after the baby is born. If your hormones are not balanced properly, you might also find yourself struggling with your weight much past the first year, along with constant headaches, mood swings, anxiety, and so much more. Often making simple changes to your diet can start the process of rebalancing your body and supporting your post-pregnancy healing.

Every mama's body is different and uses food for fuel differently. However, there are a few common things we can do that are beneficial for most, if not all, women when talking about our hormones, especially when it comes to preparing for a pregnancy, growing our babies, or healing from a recent delivery. Generally, the best, most nutritious diet for women is a higher fat (healthy fats only), higher protein diet with plenty of vegetables. This way of eating will keep our bodies fueled well, which in turns keep our hormones doing exactly what they are supposed to be doing. When we forgo healthy fats and proteins in exchange for processed snacks and nutrient-lacking meals, we are simply not giving our bodies what they need to do their jobs properly. I know this is much easier said than done, and with the exhaustion that comes from becoming a new mom, it can sometimes be overwhelming and almost un-attainable to find the time to feed our bodies what they need. This is why preparing in advance is so important.

Often, we are in such a hurry to lose the "baby weight" that we neglect adding in good-quality fats like healthy oils and avocados or nuts and seeds, as well as healthy sources of protein.

When you restrict your body from quality fats and protein, it will often have the opposite effect on you and cause your body to hang onto the weight even longer. Looking back at my previous pregnancies, I was much slower to lose the extra weight with my first four babies when I tried calorie restricting and didn't take into account the importance of proper nutrition. Once I learned to fuel my body on healthy fats, healthy proteins, and vegetables (organic whenever possible), I had no problem losing the baby weight. On top of losing the baby weight much more quickly, I found that my energy was stronger, my complexion was clearer, and I had way more focus and patience when it came to caring for my family. *And as a bonus, the only three babies that slept through the night from early on were the babies who were breastfed from a high-fat, higher protein diet. Definitely worth a try!*

On top of ensuring you're eating a healthy diet, you'll want to be sure that you are taking good quality supplements. It is always important to continue taking your prenatal vitamins that you were taking during your pregnancy well into the first year of your baby's life, especially if you are breastfeeding. Although everybody is different and nutritional requirements can vary slightly from mom to mom, I'm going to share some nutritional supplements that are very helpful both during a pregnancy and after a cesarean. These supplements can also speed up the recovery process.

A Good Quality Probiotic

Probiotics are completely safe to take during pregnancy and while breastfeeding. They help improve your immune system by balancing the good bacteria in your gut. They are especially important after your cesarean to counteract the effects of the antibiotics that they give you during surgery.

Iron

Your iron levels are crucial in preventing blood clots, keeping you strong, and supporting a healthy immune system. Making sure your iron levels are in check is vital both during and after pregnancy. Whether you're healing from a vaginal or a cesarean delivery, it's important to replace the iron that you have lost. And if you're breastfeeding, the iron supplies in your body are directly transferred to your baby to help build their liver and other vital organs. You can choose to use an iron supplement or add in high-quality food sources such as red meat and green, leafy vegetables.

Vitamin D

By now we are probably all aware that we can get a good amount of vitamin D from the sun. Vitamin D is known to absorb calcium, improve our immune systems, and protect our bones and our heart. But did you also know that Vitamin D can be an amazing tool to cheer us up? Women who are depleted in their vitamin D stores are much more likely to suffer from postpartum depression and anxiety. Taking a vitamin D supplement is an optimal choice for women who have recently given birth.

Omega-3 Fatty Acids

Omega-3s, such as DHA, play an important role for you as a new mom and will also transfer easily to your breastmilk, which is excellent for your baby. Omega-3 fatty acids are an excellent way to support both a mama and baby's brains, as well as aid in preventing inflammation and healing. They have also been found to have a positive effect on postpartum depression.

Vitamin C

Vitamin C has been proven to be an excellent source for both preventing and shortening the length of an infection. Because cesarean moms are sometimes more susceptible to infection, this is an excellent choice to add to your diet. It's also great to help prevent mastitis (a condition of inflammation or swelling of the breast that can develop in breastfeeding women), which is not fun to heal from at any time, but particularly after a cesarean. You can get additional vitamin C in your diet either from fruits and vegetables such as spinach, kale, bell peppers, and berries, or from supplementing with vitamins.

Incorporating healthy fats, good sources of protein, plenty of vegetables, and the proper supplementation for your body will put you well on your way to ensuring a positive healing experience after your cesarean. However, there is still yet another area that I feel needs some major attention: *your first BIG poop!*

Pooping after a cesarean can be absolutely ruthless! I kid you not, this is definitely something the doctors should be warning you about weeks before you head into the operating room! This is probably the most overwhelming, strenuous (literally!), and least talked about part of the entire hospital stay. No one ever seems to talk about it, and yet it is something that is pretty much required of you before they release you from the hospital. (Yes, you will likely be released if you are still struggling, but they are pretty adamant that you are either starting to poop or at least passing gas before they send you on your way!)

Because our bodies generally use a lot of abdominal muscles to pass our leftovers through our bowels, and because our abdomens, along with many other layers of tissue, have just been sliced open and then stitched back up, it's like our mind goes into a period of forgetfulness with moving things along, not to mention the pain medication we are on, the anesthetic our bodies just received, or the less-than-amazing hospital food that is definitely not designed to promote healthy digestion. It's not fun to get more and more bloated every time you eat without being able to push it all through properly. Trust me, it's painful to push, and it's painful to sit on the toilet. It is almost impossible to figure out where on earth we are expected to find the proper muscle power to get that first movement out, yet no matter what happens, we need to get that first beauty out of our body and into the toilet! And when you finally do, let me warn you in advance, *the beauty is in the size*! Your first poop may be a poop like nothing you have ever encountered before. *(Too much information? Sorry, but not sorry!)*

One of the hardest parts of pooping at the hospital is trying to find moments in the hospital room where you are not interrupted by the medical staff. *(Can we please have some privacy here!)* It seemed as though every time I would finally have a moment to myself where my baby was sleeping and I could slowly work my way to the washroom, I would immediately be interrupted by a nurse coming in for some sort of check-up or a cleaning person coming in to change the garbage. I was much too timid for my first few cesareans to say anything to the team, but as I grew in boldness for my next deliveries, I would simply let them know I was going to try to poop and ask them kindly to leave me alone for a bit longer. Nothing is worse than the moment you're finally making headway on the toilet only to have a knock on the door to shut you all down again. Be firm and let them know to come back if they find you in the bathroom.

When you're in the hospital, you'll likely be given a medicine pack for pain, which will also include stool softeners. Stool softeners definitely have their place, and it is important to stay on top of them, especially if you were not on a healthy, high-fiber diet prior to your surgery. Stool softeners help move things along by binding matter together and making it slightly softer, which in turn makes it easier for it to make an exit... eventually.

However, even more important than the stool softeners is monitoring the foods you eat leading up to your surgery and immediately following the surgery. You'll have much better luck with your first bowel movement if you've been eating healthy, high-fiber foods than you will if you've been filling up on junk food leading up to your big day. With my first two cesareans, I was not overly concerned about what I ate before my surgery. Even with the stool softeners, my first bowel movements were almost unbearable, and my stomach hurt just waiting for things to get moving. Although the stool softeners may have made the bowel movement softer, I felt it still took much longer to actually get that first poop out, which in turn led to more bloating, a sore tummy, and even pain when it was actually "go" time. With my following cesareans, I decided to try adding high-fiber foods to my diet leading up to surgery and the days immediately following as opposed to solely relying on the stool softeners the hospital provided. This made it much more enjoyable and much easier to keep things moving along.

Here are some great foods you can incorporate into your diet on the days and even weeks leading up to your cesarean if you want to make your first few bowel movements a little more pleasant! Not to mention they are full of so many vitamins and minerals that will do wonders in assisting you with both healing and breastfeeding.

Chia Seeds

Chia seeds are high in fiber, which means they will go a long way in helping you with your bowel movements during the last few weeks of pregnancy, as well as the first week following your surgery. They can relieve you of constipation while helping you excrete toxins through your bowels. They also serve as a probiotic, which is great for your digestion and improving your gut health and can also counteract some of the harm that was done from the antibiotics that they give you during surgery. Not only did I eat a ton of chia seeds during all of my pregnancies, but I also brought them along in my hospital bag to add to any food like yogurts, muffins, and soups that I ate while I was in the hospital. For me, this was the most important tool to add to my diet to help those early bowel movements without having to rely solely on stool softeners.

Hemp Hearts

Hemp hearts are another excellent choice for incorporating high fiber into your diet. They are also an excellent source of plant protein and are high in iron and zinc, which is optimal for both baby's growth and your maternal health. They are really easy to bring along in your hospital bag in addition to chia seeds and go a long way in helping your digestive track after your surgery.

Berries

Berries are loaded with antioxidants and are chalked full of nutrition that will help your body heal after surgery. They are also loaded with fiber and will help get things moving after your baby is delivered.

Avocados

I truly can't rave about these super foods enough! Whether in a smoothie, on their own, or with a bit of scrambled eggs, avocados are super helpful leading up to your surgery as well as for healing after surgery. They provide your body with amazing nutrients for breastfeeding, and they are also loaded with fiber, which again will help your bowels stay in check for your first few "poops" after surgery!

Dark Leafy Greens

Dark leafy greens are full of vitamins and minerals and are also a great source of fiber for your intestines. They'll keep things moving along nicely, so you will have a little easier time post-cesarean. They are loaded with vitamin A, C, and E, as well as vitamin K, which is so important to have after surgery to prevent blood clotting. Good sources include kale, spinach, Swiss chard, and romaine lettuce.

Basically, you want to ensure that both leading up to your surgery as well as the first few days after your baby is born you are eating foods that promote healthy digestion while also providing your body with amazing nutrients. In the end, it will make for a much easier time healing and a healthier and happier mama and baby!

Is There Anything Else I Can Do to Prepare My Body for Future Pregnancies After a Cesarean?

The foods, supplements, and choices you make during pregnancy and then as a new mom are going to go very far in ensuring that you are the healthiest version you can be. And not only will these choices help you with energy, weight, and your hormonal health, they'll also ensure you're doing the best job possible to prepare your body if you plan on having future pregnancies and cesareans.

Not every mom thrives on the same foods or diet plan; however, every mom can benefit from ensuring all of her nutritional needs are met while maintaining a healthy lifestyle. Of course, you'll want to treat yourself to some special treats after your baby is born, and you're also going to want to wait a while before starting any type of exercise routine. After all, you have just carried your little one for nine months, and you deserve some rewards. That is totally okay! Just remember that the choices you make now will have a lasting impact on your future, and both you and your baby (and future babies) deserve to have the best chance at a healthy, energetic, and positive lifestyle.

If you are like me and know you'll want more children in the future, you should start preparing as soon as possible! No, this doesn't mean a ton of extra work while you are caring for your new baby. What it does mean is that you should be aware of what you are doing to and with your body that will strengthen it again for future pregnancies.

Ever since I was a little girl, I knew I wanted a large family. There was just something inside of me that was constantly inspired whenever I envisioned a bunch of kids running around the house. I was created to be a mom, and for me, I didn't see my journey ending after three babies. It was after my third child was born—my first daughter—that my doctor came into my hospital room shortly after my cesarean to speak with me. I remember being so infatuated with my new little pink bundle and just loving on her when my doctor came in for a routine checkup. After she asked me how baby and I were both doing, she went on to discuss a few things regarding the surgery.

"Your uterus was so thin in one section that I could actually see your daughter's hair before we removed her! This definitely needs to be your last cesarean. I am so sorry. We can discuss options when you come in for your next checkup!"

Wow! I was completely shocked. As if I wasn't already hormonal enough, this was just more than I could handle hearing at the time. Although she was kind and gentle in the way that she said it, I don't truly think she will ever know how much of an impact those words had on my life at the time. I was not ready to think about this being the end of my pregnancy journey!

Needless to say, and in typical Holly fashion, I spent the next year poring over articles, books, and studies to try to figure out what on earth I could do—if anything—to build back the lining of my uterus. To my surprise, there was actually a ton that could be done! The more I researched, the more excitement I began to have about the future of my family. And even if I did not go on to expand our family size, many of the things I was learning would also be very beneficial in healing my body for optimal health and strengthening my body from the inside out.

A new spark was lit inside of me, and I became extremely passionate about healing after a cesarean. I started putting some of the techniques to work immediately, and I have continued to add them to my routine, even to this very day. I am happy to say that after all of that hard work, my doctor confirmed that the thin uterine segment was no longer a major issue after my third baby. Although not completely perfect, my doctor was okay with me going on to have further pregnancies. My doctor was still very cautious about monitoring the process during each cesarean, and I obviously have scar tissue that needs to be considered as well, but for me, just being able to dream about future babies again made all of the hard work worth it. Simply amazing!

Below I have listed for you a few extra things I have focused on or added into my life that I believe contributed to the success of my cesareans.

As always, be sure you take your doctor's advice and recommendations very seriously and include them in any future decisions. If you feel your doctor is not a good fit for you, never hesitate to get a second opinion

Raspberry Leaf Tea

If you are going to add in only one thing to your healing regimen, add this! By now, you've probably heard of all of the amazing benefits of raspberry leaf tea, and if you haven't, this is a good time to start learning. For centuries, red raspberry leaf tea has been used for many ailments, particularly those related to women's health. Because it is so rich in nutrients and antioxidants, red raspberry leaf tea offers a ton of health and nutritional benefits including reducing menstrual cramps, strengthening the uterus walls, decreasing labor time, and improving blood flow. As soon as I learned about its benefits, I was sure to add it to my daily routine! This is now something I drink almost daily, and I also supplement with red raspberry leaf capsules as needed. Because red raspberry leaves can cause mild contractions, some health-care practitioners recommend waiting until after your first trimester or even closer to your due date before you add this to your diet. Talk it over with your health-care provider in advance to make sure you are cleared to drink this tea or take the supplement. If they want you to wait, it is still something you can continue after your baby is born. If you don't like the earthy flavor of the tea, you can also drink it cold with lemon and a natural sweetener added for a refreshing iced beverage.

Improve Your Blood Circulation

Our bodies are absolutely amazing at repairing and healing themselves, but they can't do it alone. One of the most important things we need to focus on if we are attempting to rebuild our uterus lining and strengthen it so that it can both heal properly and handle future pregnancies is to ensure that our blood is circulating properly. There are so many amazing foods you can consume that will actually improve your blood circulation, which in turn helps your body repair any damage that has been caused from trauma—in my case, a very weak uterine lining and internal damage from a previous cesarean. A few of the most common blood-building and blood-circulating foods I recommend are the following:

Garlic

Along with greatly improving our immune systems and acting as a natural antibiotic, garlic is also amazing at increasing our blood flow, which in turns leads to optimal healing. The sulfur compounds in garlic cause an immediate increase to the blood flow into our tissues, making it a perfect supplement to our diets. Whether you choose to take this as a capsule or eat the cloves raw or cooked in many of your favorite recipes, garlic is definitely something you want to add to your daily routine.

High-Quality, Organic Meat

Unless your diet has other specific requirements, it's important to consume one to three servings of high-quality, organic, and hormone-free meat daily, particularly red meat. The iron provided in red meat is easily absorbed by the body, and red meat also contains a large amount of B12, which helps keep nerves and red blood cells healthy. The high levels of protein that meat offers will also help keep your bones and muscles strong, which is very important if you plan on having future pregnancies. The high iron and protein will also help directly strengthen your uterine lining by providing it with the nutrition it needs to repair itself.

Citrus Fruits

Everyone knows citrus fruit is loaded with vitamin C and is a super food when it comes to building up our immune systems. But something else that these super fruits are known for is their high level of antioxidants. Antioxidants are known to decrease inflammation, boost circulation, and help prevent blood clots. All of these go a long way in supporting and strengthening your uterine lining.

Turmeric

Increased blood flow is one of turmeric's many health benefits. According to studies published by the National Library of Medicine,[4] turmeric has been used in many cultures to both open up our blood vessels and improve our circulation. It is amazing at promoting heart health and can be a great addition to your diet either in the form of a supplement or tea.

The Importance of Exercise

During your C-section, many layers of tissue are cut and then sewn back together, which will in turn create scar tissue through multiples layers of your abdomen. This will directly affect your body's ability to properly stabilize your core. If you plan on having future pregnancies, particularly future cesareans, your abdomen will need extra time to heal and strengthen itself first. You'll want to focus on strengthening the deep muscles of your core as well as your pelvic floor.

The stronger your body is, the better chance you'll have at carrying out future pregnancies. I know how hard it can be to build

---

[4] https://www.ncbi.nlm.nih.gov/books/NBK92752/

your body back piece by piece after having a baby, especially after a cesarean, but even a few minutes a day goes a long way in helping you regain your strength. With the online world, you really don't even need to leave your house. You can find so many amazing Pilates, cardio, and strengthening videos right from the comfort of your own home that you really don't have a ton of excuses not to do it. Always be sure to look for workouts and routines that are "cesarean friendly," as many types of exercises need to be avoided after a cesarean.

The Importance of Warming Your Uterus

The uterus is truly a fascinating and powerful organ! After all, it is the only organ that has the ability to completely create a new organ—the placenta—whenever it is growing a baby. Amazing! In order for your uterus to truly thrive, it's important to create a warm environment so it can reach its full potential. Taking warm baths, applying regular castor oil packs (more on this later), and drinking nourishing teas are all simple steps you can add into your regular lifestyle that will do wonders in creating a healthy uterus for future and current pregnancies!

What Is an Appropriate Timeline for Becoming Pregnant Again?

Definitely talk with your doctor about the best timeline for getting pregnant again. Generally, they'll want you to wait at least a year after a cesarean before getting pregnant again; however, every body and each situation is unique, and your doctor may take other considerations into account before giving you the green light. And, if you find yourself like me where not all of your pregnancies were perfectly planned on the "perfect" timeline, I hope you're feeling encouraged by now that there are many things you can do to improve your chances of carrying out a healthy pregnancy and delivery!

Although you don't want to make it an obsession while healing from your cesarean, the earlier you start taking care of your body, both inside and out, the sooner you'll start seeing your body return to its new, healthy normal. Sure, it might not be exactly like it was before, but you can definitely set yourself up for many more healthy pregnancies if you make yourself a priority, too. Even taking small steps at the beginning will go a long way in healing your body in the long-term.

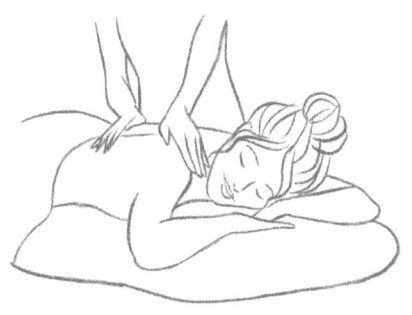

CHAPTER 14
Alternative Therapies for Healing Your Body

What can be done to prevent or heal from long-term complications of a cesarean?

NO MATTER WHAT you do to try to prevent problems during or after your pregnancy, having a cesarean unfortunately has no guarantees that you won't face future issues after your surgery. Many women experience back pain, internal issues, and problems with their scar even years into their healing journey. Luckily for us, though, there are so many alternative steps we can take that can correct these issues and ultimately restore the balance of our bodies. I always found that for me, I was most likely to have issues in my lower back, likely because my back had to work so hard to compensate for my abdominal muscles that were not functioning as they should. Even with exercising and a healthy diet, I still found that using many of the therapies below helped me regain strength in my back and heal my scar tissue much more thoroughly. Even years after your cesarean, there are many steps you can take to improve your body's ability to move, as well as heal from issues you may have dealt with for years. I have detailed my favorite alternative healing therapies that can be used to help you heal from the inside out.

Cesarean Massage

Not once during all seven of my cesarean experiences did I ever hear a doctor or nurse mention the benefit of *massaging your cesarean scar,* and yet it is one of the first things I recommend to every single cesarean mom I meet, even if it has been years since her last C-section. This is one of the reasons why I believe I was able to have so many successful cesareans with no issues with the scar tissue attaching or interfering with any of my other organs.

I first heard about scar tissue massage from a visit with my naturopathic doctor. She explained how any time we develop a scar, both externally and internally, we automatically build up a ton of extra scar tissue, which is our body's way of healing the trauma it has just been through. With a cesarean, because they cut through so many layers before even reaching your uterus, there is a lot of potential for the scar tissue to later cause lower back pain, painful urination or bowel movements, pain when having intercourse, or other varying pelvic issues. Massaging your scar can also greatly reduce the "shelf" that women often experience above their scar, especially if they have repeat cesareans.

Although you can start a cesarean massage even years after you have had your baby, the best time to start massaging your scar is as soon as you feel it is has healed externally. I usually wait about three to four weeks after my cesarean before I begin this technique. First, I gently start working on the top layer by moving the scar up and down and side to side to start maneuvering the tissue surrounding my incision. Over the next few weeks, I slowly massage deeper and deeper into the layers. Make sure you're using a soft oil such as coconut or even castor oil to help work its way into the layers. This will also help make the motion of massaging feel a bit more comfortable.

In the earliest stages of the massage, you'll want to begin by lying down and using your fingers to manipulate the skin around your incision. Even if your incision is still slightly red, you can move your fingers extremely gently around the outer area of your scar. Over the next few weeks, you should slowly be able to move directly onto your incision. You are going to feel small clusters of tissues, lumps, and areas where your incision is not as flexible as others. These are the areas that you really want to focus on. As you continue to massage into these areas, they should slowly become easier to move and less bumpy.

As you get comfortable with the first layer, you'll will want to start to apply more pressure deeper into your muscles. This may be slightly uncomfortable, but it should never cause extreme pain. If it does, then it's time to bring it back to a gentler approach with less pressure. As you move deeper into the muscle, you'll also feel areas that are clustered or perhaps tighter than others. Continue moving side to side and rotating your fingers until you feel more motion over these areas. Eventually, you'll feel these areas melt away.

Finally, you're ready to get to the deepest layer, which is the area that is closest to all of your organs and has the most potential for future problems. In order to reach this area, you'll need to be lying down again, but this time with your knees bent upwards. You'll want to apply as much pressure as you can and reach side to side deep within your abdomen. Each side should eventually feel similar, with the ability to move freely as you move this area around.

Ideally, you'll want to work on this daily until you feel you are happy with the results. Even five to ten minutes at a time can do wonders for your mobility and healing process. Even now, I still often work on massaging as a maintenance tool when I am lying down or relaxing.

Castor Oil Packs

Have you ever heard of all of the amazing benefits of a castor oil pack? When my naturopathic doctor first mentioned it to me, I have to admit I had never even heard of the term before. It honestly sounded kind of silly. However, once I learned and then applied the proper technique, I could instantly see what the big deal was. When castor oil is applied topically to the skin, it has been shown to increase circulation and improve the healing of tissues and organs. It is also a great support for your lymphatic system, which will help reduce inflammation and improve your immune system. In addition, it's a great option to help soften your scar tissue and works very well when applied after a massage. It is seriously the most relaxing thing to do after you've had a cesarean; I highly recommend you give it a try as soon as possible. Just wait until you are cleared at six weeks before you put any additional weight on your scar.

You can easily make a castor oil pack at home by using a clean, dye-free cloth that is approximately the size of your abdomen. Soak the cloth in castor oil until it's completely saturated. Once saturated, gently lay it over your entire abdomen. Then, lay a hot water bottle or heating pad on top of the cloth to activate the healing process. It is ideal to lay some Saran Wrap in between the two layers so you don't get your heating pad all greasy. Finally, lie down somewhere comfortable with this on your abdomen for twenty to thirty minutes to promote optimal healing. Castor oil packs are also a great option to use in advance anytime you feel your body is coming down with a cold or flu as it quickly stimulates the immune system, which in turn will give you a better chance at fighting the virus more quickly.

Acupuncture

Acupuncture is an excellent option when it comes to healing your body after a cesarean. Several energy channels may be interrupted during a cesarean, and acupuncture can work wonders to release these channels, which in turn can help prevent scar pain, numbness, painful menstruation cycles, and other pelvic disorders. Acupuncture has also shown great results in reducing the appearance of your scar. This is also an excellent option if you want to strengthen your body to increase the chances of having a successful VBAC or repeat cesarean.

Chiropractic and Massage

Healing from a cesarean will cause your body to rely on different muscles to do things you normally did mainly with your abdominal muscles. Your back, legs, and arms will go through a completely new workout routine just from simple movements like walking, climbing stairs, carrying your baby (and eventually the car seat), and more. Not to mention the strain on your back from the pregnancy you've just been through or all of the pressure that was applied during your surgery to pull the baby out. Our bodies go through a lot to a bring a baby into this world and even more if you are healing from a cesarean. I would never go without both chiropractic care and massage to help restore my tight muscles and align my body after delivery.

Pelvic Floor Specialists

Often after a cesarean, our midsection will feel like a wiggly bowl of jelly with very little strength from the pelvic region to the top of the abdomen. This is because you have just undergone a major abdominal surgery that sliced into many layers of skin, tissues, nerves, and muscles. If you continue to have any issues with your back, pelvic area, intercourse, urinating or bowel movements, or movement in your midsection after your cesarean, visiting a pelvic floor specialist may be something to consider. Pelvic floor specialists are trained at helping women regain strength and heal from many potential issues that can arise after a cesarean surgery. They are also an excellent option if you want to strengthen your body to increase your chances of having a successful VBAC or repeat cesarean.

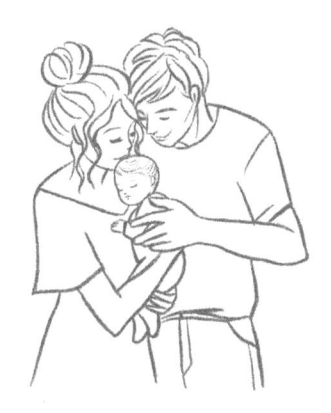

CHAPTER 15
Role of the Support Partner

How your support partner can best support you before, during, and after your cesarean.

YES, IT IS TRUE: my husband always tends to get a little squeamish on the morning of my cesarean and while watching me prepare for surgery. This isn't because he doesn't care; it's actually the complete opposite. I think it really comes down to the fact that he knows in only a few short hours he will not only witness his wife go through an overwhelming and quite scary procedure, but he'll also be introduced to another beautiful child. And although it's true that we are the ones on the operating table going through the majority of the physical toil, support partners are witnessing it all right alongside us without really being able to do anything. The entire procedure is in the hands of the medical team, and all a partner can do is wait it out. Let's make sure we give them the space they need to go through all of these emotions, too!

On top of encouraging and supporting you during the surgery, your partner also knows their role is going to be even more important than with a vaginal birth, as there will be a longer recovery period in caring for both you and the baby. As much as my husband tends to dread the physical surgery itself, he is a complete rock both during the procedure and throughout the entire healing process. He never misses a step when it comes to caring for me or for our new baby. Sometimes it's the smallest of details that makes everything else seem just a little bit easier.

There are many similarities for supporting a vaginal delivery and supporting a cesarean delivery, and this support really goes so much further than just loading the bags into the car and then waiting for Mom to have the baby. I cannot stress enough how important it is for support partners to really listen to the mom and then be an amazing advocate for her afterwards. She has just spent an entire nine months carrying this baby, and she is probably completely overwhelmed thinking of all of the things that need to get done in order to deliver this child, care for this child, care for possibly other children in the home, and then find time to heal on top of it all. It's my opinion that one of the last things that should be on a new mom's mind is having to advocate for her decisions in the hospital all alone.

A support partner who is able to listen carefully to her—even about the smallest of details—and then be her voice while she is dealing with the medical team can really lessen her burden. If she is anxious, let the team know. Thirsty? Tell them for her. If she wants to have skin-to-skin time with her baby as soon as possible, remind the doctors of that, too! Sometimes doctors and nurses are not even trying to be complacent; they are just busy doing their jobs and it's not possible to remember every single detail that was important to the mom. When a support partner is there to pass on her thoughts, fears, and questions, it can go a long way in making the situation run much more smoothly.

I am going to be completely honest with you. During all of my cesareans, I always find it way too easy to slip into a state of fear as my mind wanders off into all of the *what-ifs*. Sometimes the anesthetic can make you feel like your chest is not breathing properly. Or other times, you may catch a "look" in the eyes of one of the medical team that for whatever reason makes you feel as though something is wrong. Or at times you are completely worried about how the baby will do arriving days, possibly weeks, earlier than its original due date! It is *so* easy for your mind to suddenly fly through all kinds of disastrous possibilities, and this can steal all of your joy in an instant. Having a reassuring support partner who is constantly encouraging and advocating for you, or even passing on the tiniest of concerns to the medical team, will do wonders. You, the mom, should not have to feel as though it all falls on you. Let your support partner do the questioning and reassuring for you.

Another thing I mentioned earlier in this book was the importance of having a birth plan—and not just for you but for your support partner too. Make sure to uniquely address every item on the list with them in advance, before the big day. Don't just scan it over with them. You want to make sure that even in an emergency situation, you are on the same page with how you want this delivery to go. This will go a long way to ensure a positive experience, and it will also go a long way in making both mom and support partner feel equally a part of every aspect of this birth.

A Section Addressed to Support Partners

Everything leading up to this point has been written to you, the mama, who is undertaking an exciting, albeit sometimes intimidating, journey. Our support partners feel it, too. I've written the next section specifically for support partners. Encourage your support partner to read the message below so he or she can feel supported and understand what you may need from them during your cesarean.

As a support partner, it's very important to remember to laugh, keep things light, and enjoy the entire process. You want to make this moment as memorable for you and your partner as you can. Sure, there may be many moments where the situation calls you to be much more serious and constrained, but you will likely have many humorous and joyous moments that you'll want to make sure you are fully present for!

Caring for a new mom after the baby is born is equally, if not more, important than leading up to the procedure. Coming out of a cesarean is one to the craziest experiences she will ever have. She will likely be freezing cold, possibly nauseous, extremely emotional, elated, exhausted, hungry, dizzy, overwhelmed, full of joy, and absolutely everything in between. Continue listening to her needs and ensuring that she is receiving the best care possible. Nothing is too small or minor when it comes to making the situation feel just a little easier for the mom. Find out where the closest place to refill the ice and water are. Ask her constantly how she is feeling and if she needs anything. Don't hesitate to hold and care for the baby when she needs a break, even if it's only for a few small moments before she wants the baby back. And if she doesn't want to let go of the baby at all, that is okay, too. Sit by her side and take in all of those precious moments together.

Once she and baby are out of the recovery room and into their own beds, your role does not stop. Now is a good time to step in and help with all of the baby's needs, too. It's very difficult during those first few days post-surgery for a mom to maneuver baby around and change and dress them as needed. Everything feels exhausting and impossible. Be sure to pass baby to Mom whenever she needs and be available to change the diapers, too. So often my husband would pass me the baby so I could start feeding only to have me ask him to take the baby back immediately, so I could shift my position a little bit differently. Be available and understanding, especially in the first early days while Mom is still figuring out the groove of everything. Even when she starts feeding or snuggling baby, be available to pass her any snacks, water, blankets, or other things she needs.

Take this time to learn how to properly swaddle and care for the baby, too. If you need advice, ask a nurse. They are usually super eager to help where needed. If your partner feels like you are excited about learning and taking care of the baby too, she will likely feel much better about finding time to rest and take care of her needs.

Another important thing is to make sure that the new mom is eating well and nourishing herself during this stage. She is not able to run around finding food that gives her energy and helps her heal, yet at the same time she'll likely be very hungry with all of the new demands that have recently been placed on her body. She will have very limited options available and will eat almost anything out of desperation. This is a great time to go the extra mile: prepare her vitamins, mix some chia seeds into her yogurt, grab her some fresh fruit, or grab her the snacks she brought along in her bag as needed. Of course, you'll want to surprise her and pick up some of her favorite snacks occasionally, too. I just can't state enough how amazing it felt when my husband actually provided me with nourishing options that he picked up at home while visiting the kids or maybe at a healthier restaurant while he was going for a drive. All of these small gestures go such a long way in making the most of the hospital stay.

Once mom and baby come home from the hospital, she will likely be more tired and in more pain than she was initially. This is because the swelling and bruising from the operation really sets in, and the strong pain medication is usually out of her system at that point. Be prepared to see a bit of a decline in her energy levels. She will likely just want to rest and sit for the first few days. Be sure that you continue to bring her meals and supplies as needed, even in the wee hours of the night. She will truly heal a lot faster if she has someone who is able to do most of the running around the house for her. It is very helpful to ensure that she has everything she needs on her bedside table for those first few nights, such as medication, fresh water, snacks, lip gloss, baby supplies. While she is feeding the baby and putting him down for the night (or at least for the first sleep session), save her the extra work by gathering her the things she may need throughout the night. It is much easier to have everything easily accessible before bed than to be running around at 3:00 a.m. looking for the proper essentials.

And of course, remember to keep yourself nourished, too! Having a new baby can be extremely exhausting for both the mom and dad. Rest as often as you can as well, so that you are able to provide the best possible care for everyone. This will all be behind you soon enough, and you'll have a much better handle on everything. Mom's energy will return and within a few weeks, things will be running much more smoothly! Enjoy this time you have getting to take care of your partner and loving on your new, sweet baby. It goes by faster than you think!

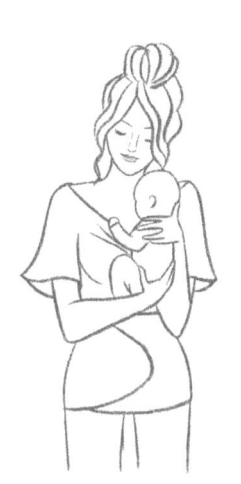

CHAPTER 16
Some Final Words

Encouragement for all cesarean moms

COMING TO TERMS with your cesarean, regardless of the reason that it happened, is going to look completely different for everyone. It is going to take time to properly grieve and then heal from a birth story that may have looked different than you expected. Learning to accept both your emotional and physical scars of childbirth may take weeks, months, or even years. That is okay! I've heard from so many moms who still feel disappointed with their birth story or are still sad that they weren't able to have the "birth" of their dreams. I understand! To this very day, I still wonder what a natural or vaginal birth might have felt like. I wonder what it would feel like if my babies came on their own time and on their own schedules. When would their birthdays be? Could I have avoided the NICU? Would I have met different people along the way? I guess some things in life are meant to be left as mysteries!

What is no longer a mystery, however, is what an amazing mom I have become! I fully know and cherish my children, and they will always call me their mom. They know how much love I have for each and every one of them. They have watched me heal from each and every one of my deliveries. They have seen me go through the pain and anxiety that comes from each birth and then embrace the love and joy that instantly follows the arrival of each new baby. They have seen my strength and my joy throughout each situation, as well as my pain and struggles. They have watched their mom grow alongside the family, learning to love and accept each and every situation as it comes—a lesson that will be much needed in their lives, too. My children have also watched me become an encourager to other moms who are going through similar situations, one of life's truly greatest gifts.

My hope is that you, too, will be able to embrace your story so that you are able to accept and cherish your baby's birth for everything that it truly is. Moms are amazing—and that includes you!

From one mama's heart to another
~ Holly

ABOUT THE AUTHOR

HOLLY FEHR is a mother of seven children, all delivered by cesarean. She is passionate about helping others fully cherish their unique birth stories, while equipping them with the proper tools and information they need to be fully prepared for their cesarean deliveries. She also loves encouraging other moms through the many stages and seasons of motherhood.

Holly lives with her husband on an acreage in Saskatchewan, Canada where she homeschools her children. In her spare time you will find her gardening, preserving food, reading, writing, and embracing life with her family. *Treasured Cesarean* is her first book.

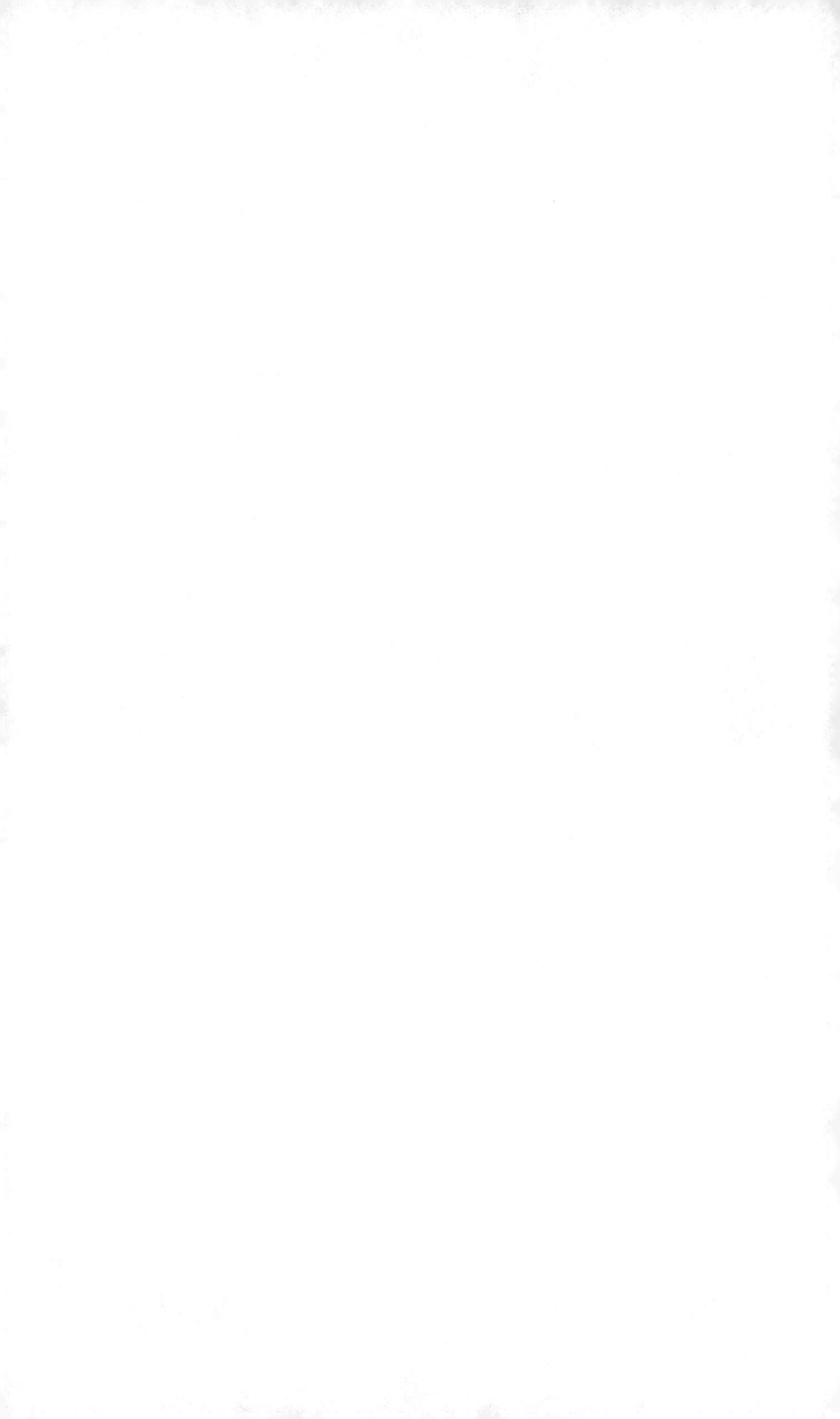

Printed in the USA
CPSIA information can be obtained
at www.ICGtesting.com
LVHW051143080224
771186LV00058B/1329

9 781039 173620